My Two-Year-Old Eats Octopus

⌘

*Raising Children
Who Love to Eat
EVERYTHING*

Published by Bull Publishing Company,
P.O. Box 1377
Boulder, CO 80306
www.bullpub.com

Library of Congress Cataloging-in-Publication Data

Piho, Nancy Tringali.
My two-year-old eats octopus : raising children who love to eat
everything / Nancy Tringali Piho.
p. cm.
Includes bibliographical references and index.
ISBN 978-1-933503-17-2
1. Children—Nutrition. 2. Food preferences in children. 3.
Food habits—Psychological aspects. I. Title.
TX361.C5P54 2009
613.2083—dc22   2009031452

CONTENTS

⌘

Contents

⌘

ACKNOWLEDGMENTS

⌘

When one's personal and professional lives merge into a project like this, there is no shortage of people who deserve to be recognized. Family, friends, work colleagues, clients and many others have all played a role in the production of this book.

My parents, Dominick and Dorothy Tringali of Columbia, South Carolina, are at the top of that list, as they have always supported and cheered on everything I've done. Thank you, Mom and Dad, from the bottom of my heart. Special thanks also to my brother John and his family, and my mother-in-law Doris Piho.

To Jim Bull, Erin Mulligan and George Young of Bull Publishing, and my agent Krista Goering: Thank you for taking a chance on me, and for your help and guidance in turning an idea into a reality.

My clients through the years at Nancy Tringali Associates, Inc., especially those at the National Chicken Council, the National Beer Wholesalers Association and Paramount Farms, Inc., motivate me to do my best. Thank you for trusting me with your work.

So many people helped me with this book by telling their stories, offering quotes, reviewing text and opening other doors for me. A big thank you for that to all my chef friends, as well as Mindy Hermann, Di-Anna Arias, Nathalie Dupree, Tania Gembala

Sechriest, Bonnie Tandy Leblang, Pam Rogers, Tom Jones, Patti Tait, Niccole de Campos, Mallory Factor, Carrie Bachman, Pat Harper, Stephen McCauley, and many others. And special thanks to Ann Limpert for her wonderful and very thorough research.

To my wonderful friends in Washington and beyond: Martha, Elaine, Sharon, Doreen, MC, Shannon, Sue, Marianne, Ivette, Emily, Susan and Betsy: Thanks for always being a phone call or e-mail away. Now can we PLEASE get together for lunch?

To my precious boys, William and Daniel, who inspired this book and continue to inspire me every day, I love you so much.

And to my Paul: Both literally and figuratively, this book would not exist without you. Thank you for the boys, for your guidance, patience and support, and for the life we've built together. And for making it all so much fun. I so look forward to our 50 years.

CHAPTER 1

⌘

"Mmmmm . . . Octopus!"

On a family vacation trip to Miami, my husband Paul, our then two-and-a-half-year-old son William, and I strolled past a Peruvian restaurant near our hotel. We stood outside for a few minutes, admiring the al fresco dining environment, perusing the menu, and prepping young Willie for the experience ahead. "Oh, look at all the good things they have to eat, Willie," we said. "Plantains! Dark beans! And lots of seafood. You love seafood!" Reassured by the presence of a highchair and a friendly maitre d', we decided to go in.

We began our meal by ordering a ceviche appetizer to share. The large platter contained calamari, octopus, and shrimp "cooked" in the traditional lemon and lime juices, along with baked plantains and a smattering of local diced sweet onions. It looked absolutely delicious.

As he had been taught (or perhaps trained) to do after so many previous experiences in restaurants, Willie asked the waiter to bring him a small teaspoon. The waiter smiled as he complied, asking, "Is he really going to eat that?"

"Mmmmm! Octopus!" Willie squealed at the first bite. "More octopus!"

His enthusiasm and delight were contagious, attracting attention and comments from diners at several nearby tables.

"I can't believe that child is eating ceviche," one grandmotherly-looking woman said. "He loves it!" her companion noted, adding, "The kids I know would never try something like that."

That comment stuck in my mind as I thought about the youngsters I am in contact with, the children who live in our neighborhood, the members of William's playgroups, and my friends' children. Why is it that so many are described tenderly as "picky eaters"? Why are so many parents afraid to try out new foods and new types of dining experiences on their kids? And, perhaps most important, why is it that people automatically assume that all children want to eat standard, mundane kid-fare, such as chicken fingers and French fries all the time?

Willie liked the ceviche, I realized that night, for the same reason that my husband and I did. It was simply good, fresh food, expertly prepared and properly seasoned. In the absence of the abundant fat, sodium, and sugar found in so many children's foods—and, indeed, in too many adult diets as well—the wonderful flavor of the seafood, juices, plantains, and onions could shine.

That evening's restaurant experience, considered with others we've had as we have introduced young William to the flavors of Indian, Vietnamese, Thai, Mexican, Greek, and many other ethnic cuisines, convinced me that my husband and I are onto something in the conscious decision we've made to *teach* our son how to eat and enjoy a wide range of foods. When Baby Daniel joined our household three years after Willie's birth, it was even more interesting to go through the food introduction process a second time. It's fascinating to compare each child's receptiveness to new foods and his different recognition and acceptance of various flavors as both grow more mature.

From our children's earliest days, we have focused on exposing them to the ideal flavor profile of individual foods. When he was about two years old, William could, by taste, identify capers, discern black olives from green, and distinguish among various types of cheese. The more exposure he has had to different cuisines, the more he has come to understand how to taste "real" foods and how their flavors contrast with foods that are run-of-the-mill, overly processed, or "flavor-enhanced" with chemical sugars or inexpensive deep-frying. As a result, we have seen him develop a happy appreciation for the joy that food can bring to one's life.

What, Me Worry?

"I found a quarter in my son's diaper. Should I be worried?"
Recent post on parenting message board

We modern-day American parents are a strange lot.

We dump the plastic baby bottles for fear of the chemical compound BPA, and we send Thomas the Tank Engine toy trains back to China at the first mention of toxic paint. We put our kids in safety helmets and water wings and coat them with layers of sunscreen. We use antibacterial soaps and gels, cringing when someone gets too close to Baby without scrubbing up first. I recently used a local e-mail list to try to buy a "gently used" car seat to have on hand in case of visitors, only to receive a barrage of e-mails warning me about the perils of buying this sort of item second-hand. Warning, warning, warning—that seems to be the buzz word of our time. From government officials and agencies to consumer organizations, scientists, and university researchers—everyone can give you a reason to steer clear, demand a recall or refund, or protest a global corporation's marketing strategies. For the most part, if the safety trend becomes big enough, we all hop on board, sometimes leaving our critical thinking skills behind.

Then there are the things that we spend money on for our kids. We invest hundreds or thousands of dollars in education, exotic travel, and more. We spend on electronic equipment, toys, sporting goods, music lessons, and trendy clothes. We dish out money for soccer teams, ballet and art lessons, and Spanish classes. We sign up our kids for many of these programs under the guise of "play-based learning." We parents will go to any length we can afford to provide "the best" for our kids.

And yet, when it comes to the foods we pump directly into our kids' bodies every day, our standards may not be the same. As a nation, our attitude regarding children's nutrition can be summed up as "whatever." We take little or no responsibility for our children's diets, instead relying largely on multinational corporations (with only nominal supervision from the federal government), whose major priority is their own bottom line, to provide products that are healthy, nutritious, tasty, and safe to eat. Oh, and we expect these products to be reasonably priced, available in every flavor and any quantity, and always accessible whenever and wherever we happen to be. The idea that what we feed our kids may not be what is best for them (or for us) is too incomprehensible, not to mention too inconvenient, to think about. Our bottom line assumption is that the corporations that feed us, and the government bodies that oversee them, all have the best interests of the customers (and their kids) at heart.

When problems do arise in our food chain, they usually make big news. Think about past scares with *E. coli* in produce and ground beef, avian flu in poultry, and Salmonella in peanut butter and tomatoes. We respond dramatically, or not at all, depending on how directly affected we are. Then, for the most part, we go back to eating, and to feeding our children in the same way that we always have. Food in this country is presumed to be safe. And for the most part, it is safe, very safe. That makes us extremely fortunate, and at the same time, very blasé. "No news is good news," we are schooled to believe.

Sometimes policies and advice do change, usually as a result of pressure from scientific and consumer groups. But it is hard to know when we can trust the information we hear. How do we know what is just a trend, and what is a sensible, long-term policy plan? Who thought much about trans fats ten or fifteen years ago? Yet in the past few years, new scientific evidence and major consumer efforts have made it so that virtually every major snack and food manufacturer in the country has eliminated the stuff as an ingredient. California recently became the first state to ban trans fats from use in restaurants, following the lead of New York City, Philadelphia, and other metropolitan areas. But, of course, the same companies that now tout their trans fat–free products were the ones that developed trans fats in the distant past to extend the shelf life of products, and then blithely marketed this artery-clogging goo for decades. It is difficult to know who should be guiding us, and whether we as consumers are making the right decisions.

It's an exciting time to be in the food world if you're a journalist or a researcher, always on the lookout for the next hot story or product. You won't be disappointed. There is something "new" all the time. But where does that leave the average American parents, who just want to feed their kids in the safest, most wholesome, nutritious, economic, tasty (and often quickest) manner possible? Shrugging their shoulders, most likely. It's hard not to develop a "How can you ever know what's really best?" resignation.

The questions I ask about the foods I feed my kids are different now from what they would have been had I not had substantial exposure to so many facets of the American food industry. Health concerns, of course, top my list, but not far behind now is another criterion that I have come to believe plays just as much of a role in separating "good" foods from "bad," and that is taste. I used to subscribe to some of the mantras of the food marketing world, such as "All foods can fit into a healthful diet." "There are no bad foods, there are only bad diets," we used to say, but I have come to see the holes in those statements. There are definitely "bad" foods—or perhaps I should say, lesser foods, as compared to more superior ones that offer us something from *either* a nutritional *or* a wonderful taste point of view, or both. Too few foods designated for, and marketed to, children offer enough of either.

It's hard to paint a picture of this situation without picking on specific food products, so I'm purposely being a little vague here. Just think about the foods and recipes that many of the kids you may know eat, or profess to like to eat, when asked about their favorites. You can find examples in virtually every food category: beverages, cereals, snack foods, entrees, sweets, and desserts. Overwhelmingly, the favorites fall into one of two categories: very sweet, or laden with fat, as in deep-fried. A third group might be heavy on the sodium, as is the case with many packaged and processed snack foods. And what else do they all have in common? At least one of two things: either a distinct lack of unique flavor, or a flavor profile that is completely warped from the way that the food tastes in its natural, prime form.

Throughout this book, I often use fruits to illustrate this point, because they are a good example of how the food industry so often takes a wonderful, natural food—such as, say, an apple or a peach—and uses it to make something else, such as a children's food product, that is of much lesser quality in terms of nutrition and taste. The sweet taste of apples and peaches is perfect in the whole fruit. But turn that fruit into "apple concentrate" or "peach concentrate" to be used as a sweetener in a multitude of kids' food products, and all you have left is sweet. The label may boast, "100% natural," and that may be true, but that label gives a false impression as to the quality of the nutritional value of the product, not to mention its flavor value.

One of the first questions I asked myself before embarking on this research and writing project was whether or not the issue of kids and eating is even a justifiable subject, given the numerous books that already exist on the topic. I asked myself whether and why the topic merits yet another book. After all, you could say that hunger alone solves a lot of the standard eating problems. And by the time most of these kids reach adulthood, they, like most of us, will have learned to navigate their way well enough through grocery stores, kitchens, and restaurants to feed themselves sufficiently. The answer to the question about the relevance of picky eating at a young age depends on whom you ask, or perhaps from which angle you look at the topic.

It's easy to see the need for such a book from a medical perspective. With 13% of American children ages two to five overweight or obese, and another 18% of kids ages six to eleven in the same category, there is no question that childhood obesity is a serious public health problem. With regard to specific nutrients, what kids eat is also a real problem: once-conquered diseases such as rickets, caused by a lack of vitamin D, are presenting again in children, as are illnesses resulting from iron deficiencies.[1]

And how important is the psychological role that food plays in the parent-child relationship? I provide food for you; you eat for hunger, nourishment, and then enjoyment. Later you stop eating as a way to gain my attention, punish me when you feel controlled, or just to test me in an effort to learn about boundaries and limits. Out of guilt, embarrassment, or exhaustion, I give in and give you what you *want* to eat, rather than what you *should* eat, or what the rest of the family is eating. You respond by eating too much or too little. This goes on for weeks or months or years, shaping or reflecting a distorted relationship.

Theories and strategies about what to do with kids who have eating problems, real or imagined, abound. As I was working on this project, two best-selling cookbooks advocating methods of sneaking healthful foods into standard kids' recipes were much-talked-about in many parenting circles. "Acknowledging your kids' genuine (food) dislikes without being confined by them" is the message here, as these authors scheme to hide pureed vegetables in recipes for pancakes, brownies, muffins, and other favorites. The amount of clamor these books instigated, both positive and negative, reinforces the idea that feeding is a front-burner issue for many parents.

In sorting out all of this, I became convinced that there is indeed room for discussion about kids and eating from one point of view that is often overlooked. That point of view is the role of the taste of kids' foods.

What This Book Is, and What It Is Not

This book is not written to be a guide to children's nutrition, a medical discussion on the health benefits of a proper diet, another discussion on the perils of childhood and adult obesity, or a parenting primer with advice on handling the inevitable conflicts that arise as young children are being trained to sit at a table and eat a meal. I'm not a doctor or any sort of health professional, nor am I a researcher or even a professionally trained chef. What I am is a mother of two little boys, the wife of a real "super taster" who loves good food and drink, a fairly accomplished home cook, and a public relations professional who has worked for almost twenty years in the food industry.

In my business, I have come in contact with a lot of chefs. I know restaurant trends, grocery store layouts, new food products, cookbook authors, and many people in the food media. I have worked for numerous food companies and industries, including chocolate, chicken, candy, beer, pistachios, farm-raised salmon, fruits and vegetables, sugar, and dairy products. I've practiced enough to know how to pull together a simple-but-tasty dinner party. I've learned much about nutrition from working on programs, such as 5 A Day for Better Health, with organizations, such as the American Dietetic Association, and with prominent doctors and dietitians. I've taken numerous cooking classes and have grown to appreciate and advocate the seasonal and local concept of food choice, particularly with produce. I've absorbed much about the business side of the food industry from my clients, have studied up on food safety, and have even had some exposure to regulatory and federal government lobbying concerning agricultural industry issues. In short, for all of my professional life, I had been immersed in various facets of the U.S. food industry, not as an expert in any one area, but with a comprehensive knowledge broader than that of the average person.

And then I had children. And with real people that I love and am responsible for feeding on a daily basis, the situation suddenly became a lot clearer to me. People don't eat trends, nutritional components, units of perishable parts, SKUs, dietary guidelines, phytosterols, vitamin compounds, recipes, further-processed-versus-fresh products, or any of the other concepts and buzzwords that reflect an invisible barrier that exists between farmers, manufacturers, chefs, and other industry producers and the final consumer in modern-day America. We eat food.

To some of us, or to all of us at some point in our lives, that means nothing more than satisfying our urges from one hunger pang to the next, with cost or convenience being the only factor determining choice. To others, food is a political statement or a nutritional mandate, chosen carefully to reflect personal views or to fortify the body's physiological needs. To the stressed or depressed, food is a comfort item or a consoling friend; to the modern-day epicurean, food is a constant source of self-satisfaction. We can take for granted in this country that the foods that we like to eat are safe for us to eat (even if not particularly good for us to eat), and that they will be available when we want them.

By the time most people reach adulthood, the process by which they select foods each day, be it a healthy or an unhealthy one, is purely rote. We may think a little about preferences (Chinese or Mexican tonight?), stop to appreciate a wonderful food aroma or sight (Gosh, that smells (or looks) good!), or suddenly realize that it's 3:00 in the afternoon, and we'd better grab something to eat because we're "starving." But serious thought about the food we choose each day? No time, thanks.

However, when you have children, a new dimension is added. You realize the power of your influence as parents, and you know that you have just a few fleeting years to influence (or limit) your children's thought processes in a way that will serve them for the rest of their lives. A reasonable question then becomes: what, exactly, do we want to teach our kids about food, this thing that is so critical to our very existence?

Like so many other aspects of our being, our palates, our sense of taste, and our recognition of and appreciation for flavors are *developed* over the course of our lives. This sounds so simple, but it is actually quite interesting if you stop to think about it: babies must be taught not only the physical steps of how to eat, but what to eat, first from the perspective of safety, then for health, and finally for pleasure and enjoyment. There is mounting evidence that we as parents can influence these choices even before a child's birth, and certainly by our own actions during their formative years.

So how should we be using that influence? What kind of eaters do we want to produce? I can't speak for everyone, but I do know enough people who want to raise children who grow up to have healthy, positive, and pleasurable attitudes toward food and eating that I believe there must be a lot of us out there. To that end, in this book I lay out some positive, concrete steps you can take to raise a little person who will grow into an adult with a good relationship toward food.

As with most childrearing tasks, this can be a long, slow process, one that often seems to move you two steps forward and then one step back. You will no doubt encounter numerous potential pitfalls and some inevitable setbacks along the way. The eventual goal—raising an adult who can appreciate food from social, economic, health, and emotional points of view—is far in the distance and seems to have little to do with your present-day four-year-old who is whining for French fries—again. But read this book with an open mind, make a little bit of effort, and I bet you'll be surprised at some of the tangible results you will begin to see; small at first, perhaps, but moving your family in the right direction nonetheless. Just be sure to recognize these little victories: a child whose face lights up when eating an in-season strawberry or homegrown tomato, or who demands Grandma's stuffing at the Thanksgiving dinner table, or even one who actually advocates, in the presence of his friends, a visit to a new ethnic restaurant rather than a chain place. Children who make small steps like these are on the path to discovering the joy that food can bring to life.

In writing this book, I interviewed many chefs across the country. When I spoke to these certified food pros, I was struck by how many of them came from what they described as "non-food-loving backgrounds." A very significant number said that they grew up in homes where mom always cooked, and that, in many cases, her cooking was, well, not exactly top-notch. Many chefs mentioned that their childhood diets were composed of "vegetables from a can" or "a basic meat-and-potatoes diet." Still, somewhere along the way, these chefs developed an interest in food, enough to pursue it and make it a career. Many spoke almost reverently and with perfect recollection of a wonderful cook, a special meal, or a certain food that they encountered at some point that provided a life-changing experience with regard to what they ate. And now, having discovered this world of "good food," they are eager that their own children should not miss out on one of the simple joys of life. Almost all of them said that they want their own kids to start "loving food" (though not necessarily cooking professionally) from a young age.

I also interviewed numerous health professionals: medical doctors, dietitians, scientific researchers, psychologists, and others who are more educated than I am, especially when it comes to issues concerning the human body. I read an inordinate amount of medical research and published scientific literature. Naturally, I noted that their interest in the topic of "children and eating" comes more from a health and nutritional well-being standpoint than from a pleasure point of view. Combining these various perspectives became the goal of this project.

There will be points in this book with which some parents, educators, and even medical professionals will not concur, and there will be some points that will not apply to all children.

If mealtime is a constant battle at your house, for example, and you sense that your children have figured out how to use food and eating as manipulation tools, then there may be more serious discipline or psychological problems that need to be addressed before the goals of taste exploration and simple enjoyment can be achieved. Food allergies can also prevent the implementation of some of these eating strategies. Although this is a very serious concern for many parents, it's one I don't address here, primarily because of my lack of medical qualifications. And throughout the writing of this book, I have been repeatedly reminded about the child who, for years on end and for whatever reason, is simply not interested in his food, or just doesn't seem to care much what he eats. If you have a child like this, help him or her embrace other good points! Despite parental preferences, he or she just may not be cut out to be a "foodie." I'm convinced that the real number of children that fall into that category is small, however. After all, most children are interested in what we present to them as "interesting."

You'll also notice that I've focused this book on the eating habits and palate development of young kids, from newborns up to age five or six. Elementary school–age children and middle-schoolers, not to mention teenagers, can have their own eating and food issues, but those are beyond the scope of this book. I've focused on this youngest age group for a couple of reasons. For one thing, I am convinced that many habits concerning eating are formed in the very early years, so I think more attention needs to be paid to the little guys and girls and how they learn to eat. And since my personal experience as a parent has only taken me to the preschool level, I can't offer much advice for the more sophisticated eating problems that may arise in older kids. At the end of each chapter, I've summarized the advice and tips I've learned about each stage of child eating and feeding, from both the experts and my personal experiences.

This book is not for people who are looking for a sure-fire method to turn little Alex or Amanda into a gourmet or even a perfect guest at a neighbor's cookout or birthday party. I can't promise that your kids will ever love to cook with you, grocery shop with you, or behave well when they eat out with you. I'm also not writing this book for the many good parents who will see no point in all of this; some people have other priorities about what they want to teach their kids, and as long as they don't go hungry and they consume a relatively balanced diet, these people have limited concern about what their kids eat. And that's fine with me; I'm making no judgments about how you choose to raise your kids or what you want to teach them. As parents today, many of us feel pressured enough to protect our kids, school them in our values, and educate them adequately to assume their role in the world. For some people, food choice, palate development, and the ins and outs of good food just don't rank highly enough on the scale of priorities in life to merit this kind of attention.

But there are many other parents and caregivers out there who are very interested in this issue, for any number of reasons. Some of these reasons are quite practical: there is no doubt that it is simply easier to be with children who are "good eaters," whose pickiness does not dictate what or where everyone else must eat, and who do not require the preparation of a separate meal every time you leave the house.

Maybe you're a new parent with a young child or two, and you'd like to know whether the food rebellion problems you've seen in other people's kids can be prevented, or at least curtailed, by taking some proactive steps early on. Maybe you're aware of the studies that indicate food preferences established in childhood often persist throughout life, and you want to give your kids a leg up in this area. Or perhaps you already have some young Picky Eaters at your house, and you're hoping that some bad habits can be reversed. (They can be!)

Or maybe it's just that you're a real food lover yourself, and you think it's important to pass along to your children the real joys that food can bring to one's life. Food lovers are people who think that part of the fun of travel to a new neighborhood or city or country is seeking out a special restaurant or eating opportunity; people who want to teach their kids that there is nothing better, really, than sitting down to a delicious meal with family and friends, that perfect asparagus and strawberries are the true harbingers of spring, or how good the first peaches of summer will be once you make them into a golden peach cobbler. It is for you who share these goals that I offer these thoughts on broadening kids' food horizons. I hope that you find them helpful!

CHAPTER 2

⌘

So What's the Problem?

I f you're the parent of a young child, you know someone like this. In fact, it may even be you: the mom or dad who is completely beholden to a youngster's eating preferences, whims, and mandates. An entire family can be affected, as this child becomes the pint-size decider or veto vote on where to eat out or on a new recipe to try. "We always eat at (insert name of any national restaurant chain); it's the only place that has something all of the kids like," a parent will say, as if his or her own opinion doesn't matter. The child who is a picky eater is so expected, so normal, so catered to, that having one in the family hardly rates high on the list of most parents' concerns. "But he's healthy." "That's what vitamins are for." "At least he's eating something." "She'll grow out of this as she gets older," some parents rationalize.

Well, maybe, and maybe not. How often do you hear about a teenager who suddenly becomes an adventuresome eater? But even if yours is one who does develop an interest in food in her teens or later, how does that help the toddler or young child situation today?

Stories from parents about kids and eating—usually about someone else's kid, and his or her eating—abound. Chef Bob Waggoner of Charleston Grill in Charleston, South Carolina, a Los Angeles–bred chef who discovered the joys of food while living in France and now applies these cooking techniques to classic southern Low Country fare, tells of going to a neighborhood potluck Halloween party "where everyone brought something, and there were piles and piles of food, so many different things." Yet, the mother of one seven-year-old boy took one look at the table, announced that "there is nothing here that my son will eat," and asked the hostess if she could go into her kitchen "to find something that he will be comfortable with."

A mom told me about a neighborhood parent calling before a birthday party to get detailed information on the food to be served, and then sending her son over with his own bag of treats. "He wants to be sure that his Popsicle is purple," she explained. I heard lots of tales of kids who show up at friends' houses, church events, and sleepovers carrying bags of fast food, not wanting to risk actually having to eat something that is unfamiliar. There are many kids who seem to have grown accustomed to personalized catering.

Lynne, a Washington, D.C., mother of a four-year-old and a two-year-old, tells the story of a recent Christmas dinner at her house, to which she invited three other couples who also had children about the same age. She planned a nice dinner that included a salmon appetizer, followed by filet mignon, roasted potatoes, and a vegetable. "But what are the kids going to eat?" one of the other mothers asked. Rather than expect her three-year-old twins to enjoy the meal with the rest of the group, this mother brought along string cheese, grapes, and yogurt to feed her own children. "And so for Christmas dinner, they had the same thing that they eat every other night of the week," Lynne said.

And Angie, a Houston-area mother of three school-age children, told me about a vacation to Alaska that she, her husband, and their kids took with another young family. A self-described "restaurant nut," Angie had spent a lot of time online before this particular trip, researching ideal dining spots. She just assumed that the other parents—good friends whom she and her husband thought they knew so well—would want to take their own kids out, too, to enjoy new dining experiences in this exotic locale. Angie said that she learned the hard way that good friends don't necessarily make compatible travel companions, as the other parents "seemed terrified at the idea of giving their children anything to eat that might be unfamiliar to them."

"I mean, there we were on a once-in-a-lifetime trip to Alaska," Angie recounts, "an area with some of some of the best seafood in the world. And this mother—my friend—insisted on stopping at Wal-Mart to pick up things to make peanut butter sandwiches to take to the restaurants so that her kids 'wouldn't have meltdowns' when they saw the strange food."

"Enough!" you may be saying. "Enough of these bratty kids and their parents, who need to worry more about discipline and less about pasta versus osso bucco." And there is certainly something to that: everyone, from child psychologists, to grandmas, to chefs who expect their own kids to enjoy various foods, to your pediatrician, to the know-it-all mom or dad next door, will tell you that children's food issues can either start as, or quickly deteriorate into, discipline and control issues.

At some point, we've all given in to a child's food preference, simply out of fatigue, embarrassment over a tantrum, laziness, or misplaced personal guilt, or because we just don't want to fight that particular battle at that particular time. But what is the line between "at some point" and making this a constant way of life that actually rewards the child's picky eater behavior?

To gain a better understanding of the Picky Eater, make it a point to observe children. The next time you're out in a large public gathering spot, such as a shopping mall or airport, take a look at the kids in the crowd, especially the stroller-set. The majority will be snacking on something or will have some sort of food stowed in a bag so that it's readily available: a box of apple juice, a bag of pre-packaged cookies or crackers, or candy of some sort. Older kids might be toting a soft drink. Go to any family-type restaurant with young children in tow, and watch how fast the hostess will automatically hand you a "children's menu," along with the booster seat and box of crayons. The contents of the children's menu? You can recite it by heart: chicken fingers, cheeseburger, hot dog, pizza, grilled cheese sandwich, spaghetti or other pasta, peanut butter and jelly sandwich.

Standard snacks during nursery or preschool breaks? Cheesy "fish" crackers or graham crackers and apple juice. And during visits to the bank, barber shop, or other neighborhood store, even when checking into hotels or stopping by a rental car counter when traveling, well-meaning merchants will ask: "Can I give him a lollipop or other candy?" (At least most of these people ask permission first!) Julia, a mother of three, told me that her young sons are particularly adept at ferreting out the specific adults whom they know will slip them cookies or other goodies at neighborhood gatherings and such, "even after I've said no to something."

In 2002, Gerber Products Company conducted a large national study on the feeding patterns and eating habits of infants and toddlers. For five months, researchers monitored and observed more than 3,000 children ages four months to twenty-four months, representing diverse geographic, socio-economic and ethnic dimensions of this country, to determine what they ate or were fed on a daily basis. Results of the study have been released in several formats since, the most recent being a 2006 *Time* magazine special report called "Eating Smart."

The results of the study are not surprising; we learn again that kids are eating too many calories, too much sodium, and too many foods that lack substantial nutrients. Up to a third of these children consumed no fruits or vegetables, unless you count French fries. What may be surprising, however, is the extent of this problem and the age at which it now starts. From the results of this study, it appears that so-called kid foods, such as French fries, hot dogs, sweetened fruit juices, and candy, are really toddler foods, as they make up the bulk of the diet for many children who have yet to see their second birthday. Some statistics from the survey:[2]

♦ Seven percent of children *9 to 11 months old* eat French fries *every day*. In the 19 months to 2 years old category, that figure grows to 25% of children.

♦ *Sixty percent of one-year-olds* eat dessert or candy *every day*. Sixteen percent add a daily salty snack to the menu. And by the time children are 19 months old (that's just over a year and a half, when most children aren't even talking yet), 70% are consuming daily sweets, and 27% a salty snack.

♦ Thirty to forty percent of children just 15 months old consume a fruit drink (which is, by the way, primarily sugar) every day. Ten percent are already daily consumers of soda.

♦ One-quarter (25%) of children 18 months to 2 years old eat hot dogs, sausage, or bacon every single day.

A 2007 study by the National Center for Health Statistics showed that tooth decay in the baby teeth of children aged two to five is on the rise, a trend largely attributed to increased amounts of sugar consumption. "(Parents) are relying more on fruit snacks, juice boxes, candy, and soda," says the author of the study.[3]

The negative health implications of these dietary trends at such a young age are ominous, according to pediatricians and dietitians who study public health. But leaving the medical issues to the health professionals, consider another important issue. If kids are feasting on a steady fare of these foods, it seems obvious that it is at the expense of other foods that could add variety to the diet. And if parents look at these as "default foods" that they know will satisfy their kids' appetites, you can pretty much bet that they are not making much of an attempt to introduce other foods of varying colors, textures, and flavors to the routine. Behold, the Picky Eater is born.

"But I Don't Like That"

"Be sure to toast the bread for Ben's sandwich, and then cut the crust off. He likes Swiss cheese and mayonnaise—no mustard—but only on one piece of the bread. And Annie will eat some of that pasta we had for dinner last night, but it needs to be reheated to a lukewarm temperature and you have to scrape the parsley out of it. Give whatever is left over from their lunch to the dog."
A mom's instructions to a baby-sitter

Toddlers, children, and adolescents who display picky eater traits do so across a wide spectrum. And like many stages that occur in childhood, these can wax and wane, sometimes appearing and passing as a phase, others developing into long-term habits.

Some Picky Eaters are relatively easy to live and eat with. They may be generally receptive to trying some new foods, while maintaining an ongoing list of definite refusals. Their particular list of "I won't eat thats" may be annoying—foods mixed together, for example, or anything spicy, or anything green—but not too limiting in the big scheme of things. Other kids are the stuff of legends—the children who routinely drive their parents so crazy over the issue of food that mom and dad give up entirely and let them eat whatever they want, whenever they want it.

Many others fall somewhere in the middle, displaying a pickiness that comes across almost as a quirkiness. These are the kids who won't eat an apple that isn't peeled, for example, or toast that is too brown or not brown enough. They're fine with baked potatoes and sweet potatoes, but won't touch boiled potatoes. We attended a weekend house party at the beach once, and several of the young kids went through the many boxes of cereal available, picking out just the items in the granola mix that they wanted to eat and discarding the rest.

Green grapes are in; red grapes are out. A certain brand of lunch meat, day after day. Chicken is fine, as long as it has the skin off (or on), is a white meat (or dark meat) piece, and is fried or grilled (or baked or stir-fried). And on and on. As long as you can keep track of it all, you can probably get enough calories and nutrients into these Picky Eaters for them to sustain a healthful diet. For many parents, that is enough. The kids will eventually grow up and be responsible for their own food choices. Then they can either carry on with this finicky eating, or adapt to more adult-like options. It's not worth the battling now, their parents say.

Except when you and your kids are eating out or are at someone else's house, and they "can't find anything to eat." Or on one of those (perhaps rare) days when you have the time and are interested in trying something new in the kitchen, and you realize that there are so many items that your child won't eat that it's not worth the trouble. Or you have a child who begins to get a little pudgy, or perhaps too thin, or suffer from another ailment as the result of a diet that is not varied enough to provide a broad base of nutrients. These are the moments that make the picky eating problem glaringly obvious.

Teaching vs. Tricking

"The parents I know end up sticking with the tried and true—white pasta, peanut butter and jelly sandwiches, macaroni and cheese, chicken nuggets, and pizza—only because these foods are generally eaten without a fight."
Missy Lapine in *The Sneaky Chef*. Running Press Publishers, 2007

"I have become an expert at hiding vegetable purees—foods my kids wouldn't touch otherwise—in all their favorite dishes."
Jessica Seinfeld in *Deceptively Delicious*. Harper Collins, 2007

You may be familiar with prominent family cookbooks that espouse the "sneak it in" method of cooking. These writers contend that their own children refused to eat healthful foods, such as vegetables, until they, as smart moms, devised a way to trick their offspring into doing so. The books contain page after page of recipes for kid-friendly dishes, including brownies, mozzarella sticks, quesadillas, chocolate chip cupcakes, and more. The surprise, however, is that all of the recipes for these popular dishes contain purees of vegetables, such as squash, spinach, carrots, cauliflower, and broccoli. There are many advocates of this system to "trick" young children into eating healthful foods that they would find "disgusting," were they to face them directly on the plate.

While this practice may work as a method to "fool" children into eating a little bit more of what is good for them, I do have serious reservations about the message that this sends to kids, and what it ultimately teaches them about their food. Most obvious: what, exactly, is wrong with the taste of vegetables? Why shouln't young children be taught or expected to eat a carrot for the carrot's sake? Why would we ever want to think that vegetables can or should taste like dessert?

To gain first-hand knowledge of this eating strategy, I read two of the most popular of these books from cover to cover and prepared a number of recipes from each. My honest appraisal of the recipes, overall: while some kids may like them (Willie was lukewarm on most of them; baby Daniel liked them better), for the most part, the taste and nutritional end result don't justify the considerable time required to prepare them. The sweets and desserts, especially, fell into the "not worth it" category. And all of them had very little, if any, adult appeal. Most of these recipes are very kid-oriented, featuring a supposedly healthier version of things that you would find on any children's menu or in any children's cookbook—macaroni and cheese, chicken nuggets, sloppy joes, meatballs, fish sticks, and pigs-in-blankets.

"These books promote gastronomic regression," writes noted food journalist Raymond Sokolov in his *Wall Street Journal* column "Eating Out." "They re-introduce their targets' tastebuds to baby food." Sokolov himself sampled a macaroni and cheese dish from each book and called the recipes "low-end distortions of a classic dish that do not help the girl or boy at the receiving end evolve into a grown-up eater." Indeed.

And what about the confusion factor? "If you add spinach to brownies at home, how do children understand that not all brownies are created equal?" writes award-winning registered dietitian Annette Maggi, a Minneapolis author. "The brownies at school, the brownies at a friend's house, the brownies sold at a

C-store—kids will be raised to believe these are an okay snack because they look just like the ones made at home. No one said it was necessarily easy, and yes, kids can be picky eaters, but if kids aren't taught to enjoy the multitude of flavors of foods, as well as taught that eating a variety of foods leads to good health, what will their eating habits look like as adults?"

"I think the whole concept destroys a child's burgeoning food consciousness," New York–based writer and parenthood.com food columnist Larissa Phillips added. "If you are supposed to eat brownies on certain occasions and eating them makes you feel a certain way, and spinach is part of something else entirely, why would you confuse children by combining the two and present- ing them as one in the same? I also want my kids to develop an instinctive sense of where you get the various nutrients your body is asking for. If you body wants calcium or iron, like you'd find in spinach, do you provide that by eating a brownie?"

Adds cookbook author and food writer Monica Bhide, "I don't hide food from my kids; I show them what I'm doing. I don't want them growing up thinking that the only way to eat peas is to have them pureed inside some soup. I have no restrictions from my kids. I don't hide ice cream or candy from them. If my son wants candy, he comes and asks for it. The only thing I do restrict is *portion* sizes. He can have a little piece of candy and that's OK but that's it."

It seems to me, too, that, as well-intentioned as this idea may be, "sneaking" and "deceiving" kids, tricking them into eating certain foods, is the wrong approach altogether. They're pretty smart little creatures, you know, and will one day wise up to the game. Then what? You will have on your hands an even older child who will be inexperienced in tasting vegetables, and who has been conditioned to think that they must *really* be awful because they had to be hidden.

Better to focus on working with and perhaps trying to remedy the picky eater problem, maybe even before it starts.

So to begin with: How did we get into this situation in the first place? Is it just in some kids' nature, or is it the way that we nurture? Or some combination of the two?

The Big Three

One thing that we can say for certain: children's diets, like those of many other Americans, contain too much of what I refer to in this book as the Big Three: Fat, Sodium, and Sugar. At least 30% of the calories in the average child's diet are derived from sweets, soft drinks, salty snacks, and fast food, writes Marion Nestle, PhD, MPH, in a 2006 article on childhood obesity in *The New England Journal of Medicine*.

It's ironic, in a way, that the Big Three have wreaked so much havoc on Americans' health and diets, because they are three flavors that we are bred through nature to seek out and prefer. Enough fat in the diet ensured our survival through those cold Ice Age winters and helped us to absorb fat-soluble vitamins and minerals. Salt, ingested in proper amounts, helps to maintain body fluids and prevent dehydration, important because early humans spent a lot of time in motion. And a preference for sweet over bitter and other harsher-tasting flavors is said to have prevented us from ingesting many a poisonous plant in the wild. So none of the Big Three is inherently "bad," it's just that in modern-day America, and particularly in terms of how we feed our kids as a nation, we've gone way overboard.

"An unhealthy diet can lead to an unhealthy child," says Mindy Hermann, RD, a prominent health and nutrition writer and the mother of two teen-age sons. "Kids who eat a lot of foods that are high in calories but low in important nutrients may be on the road to excess weight, diabetes, and other illnesses."

"I prepare just about everything for my kids with mostly fresh ingredients, and now my boys don't like many packaged foods because they find them too salty," she added. "The fat issue is an interesting one, too. Packaged foods often have a lot of calories in a small portion because of their relatively high fat content, and they don't fill my boys up. It's much better if I make them something that has less fat and more food."

Overindulgence in fat, sodium, and sugar is one of the causes of the obesity epidemic that is gripping our country, Hermann added. Of course, a lack of exercise and increasingly sedentary lifestyles play a big role, too, but it is what we put in our mouths, and in what amounts, that is the biggest culprit in this rising public health crisis.

So here they are, with a little more information about the proper and improper roles that they play in our diet—a quick rundown on the components of the Big Three.

FAT

For all the bad press it gets, fat is an essential nutrient. Our bodies need it to absorb fat-soluble vitamins and minerals, so it is beneficial in limited amounts. The problem comes when too much fat, particularly of the wrong kind, is consumed.

Fat is the most "fattening" (pun intended) nutrient that we eat, providing nine calories per gram consumed. Contrast that to the four calories per gram provided by carbohydrates and proteins. It's also the stuff that gives many foods a wonderful mouth-feel and makes them taste richer. It may be why you prefer buttered popcorn to plain, or a luscious steak to a lean boneless chicken breast. A good example of fat's role in kid-food production is the oil used to deep fry French fries and chicken nuggets.

It's important to remember that there are three kinds of fat. Two kinds of fat are found naturally in foods: saturated and unsaturated. A good way to tell them apart is to remember that saturated fats—found in such products as butter, red meat, and lard—are solid at room temperature. They come primarily from animal products. Unsaturated fats, derived from plant products, are liquid at room temperature. They include vegetable (peanut, canola, olive, sunflower, corn) oils and the oils in nuts, seeds, and many fish.

Consumption of saturated fat is the major cause of high cholesterol levels, so these should have only a small place in the diet. Unsaturated fats are the ones that you may have heard referred to as the "good" fats; if they replace the "bad" fats in the diet, they may help to reduce blood cholesterol levels.

Even less healthful than saturated fat is the third kind of fat: trans fat. This is the type of fat that you really need to watch out for. Trans fats are mainly manufactured (as opposed to natural) fats and are typically listed on the ingredient labels of many processed foods as "partially hydrogenated oil" of some kind. It is recommended that you eat—and allow your children to eat— as little of this type of fat as possible, as overconsumption is directly linked to diseases, especially coronary heart disease. You'll notice that many processed foods now proudly tout a "No trans fats!" label; of course you must keep in mind that just because something is now trans fat–free does not necessarily make it suddenly healthful. Many fried and baked goods, as well as snack foods, are still unhealthful in large quantities, even without the trans fats. Processed foods that are "trans fats–free" (or "sugar-free," or "low in sodium," for that matter) can still be calorie-dense and nutrient-free.

SODIUM

Sodium is a mineral found in the salt shaker on your table, naturally in almost all foods (especially meats and cheeses), and also, in much higher quantities, in pre-packaged, processed foods that you buy. Salt is often used for preservation purposes, and it's also what makes potato chips, bacon, cold cuts, salted seasonings, fast food, and many condiments appealing. Who among us doesn't have a "salt craving" from time to time? But our bodies actually need very little of this mineral to function effectively—about 250 milligrams per day, which is easily obtained if you only eat natural foods. To show you the level of our salt addiction, the U.S. Dietary Guidelines allow adults up to 2,400 milligrams per day, about the equivalent of one teaspoon of salt. The average American, however, takes in 4,000–6,000 milligrams per day; in Asian countries, it's more like 8,000 milligrams. For kids, the recommended amount is lower: no more than 1,000 milligrams per day for children age 2–3, and 1,200 milligrams per day for those ages 4–8.

Have you ever seen someone pick up a salt shaker and salt food, before even tasting it? That is because people get used to the level of salt that is typically in their diets. If you eat a lot of salty foods, processed foods, or condiments, then less-salty foods will taste too bland. It also works the other way: if you are used to foods in their more natural low-salt form, then many packaged, processed, and overly salted foods will taste too salty. The message here is that we need to watch the salt intake and use it in moderation to help kids' taste buds learn to recognize and accept a healthful level of salt in their diets.

More than a quarter of the salt in our daily diets—and 80% of the total U.S. sodium consumption—typically comes from processed foods. Salt is relied on very heavily in American processed food manufacturing. And this is one important point to remember about salt: it is generally not the salt that is added by chefs and home cooks to their *properly seasoned* recipes that causes the problem. ("Salt shaker" salt makes up only about 11% of the total amount that we eat.) Salt, used correctly and in moderation, is an important ingredient in recipes because it draws out and enhances the natural flavors of the individual ingredients. If you avoid packaged and processed foods to the greatest extent possible, as well as fast foods, then you most likely will not have a problem with excess salt in your diet, even if you reach for the salt shaker on occasion.

SUGAR

What to say about sugar? We all know it and love it, and we have probably since birth, as "sweetness" is the first flavor that babies experience in mom's milk or formula. Sugar is one of the two carbohydrates (the other is starch) that we need in our diets for energy, and there are, of course, several kinds of sugar. Sucrose is the white stuff that you think of when you hear the word "sugar." Fructose is the natural sugar that is in fruits; it's why peaches, bananas, and strawberries are sweet. Lactose is another natural sugar that lends its sweetness to dairy products, such as milk. And glucose is the sugar found in wheat-based products, such as breads, pastas, and cereals.

Some form of sugar is in just about everything we eat, both naturally and as additives. High-fructose corn syrup (HFCS) is a good example of the latter; since the 1970s, when it was first developed, HFCS has been the sweetener of choice added to sodas and most packaged and processed goods. Made from corn, it's relatively cheap to produce and use, and it does a good job in extending the shelf life of products. As far as taste goes, its sweetness quotient is almost exactly on a par with "real sugar" (sucrose). It's important to mention this because Americans now consume more HFCS than they do actual sugar. Check the labels on your packaged food boxes and cans sometime; you may be surprised to see the extent to which HFCS is used.

So there you have a quick description of each of the elements of the Big Three. Technically, I should not include the word "sugar" in this group, because, as just stated, it is really other manufactured sweeteners—not only other sugars, such as high-fructose corn syrup, but also artificial sugar substitutes, such as aspartame (Nutra-Sweet), sucralose (Splenda), and saccharin—rather than sucrose that are a big part of the sweet-tasting foods and beverages that we consume. So to be precise, the Big Three are Fat, Sodium, and Sweeteners. But since that doesn't roll off the tongue quiet as smoothly, and most people are more familiar with the word Sugar, I will continue to label the Big Three as such.

It may seem that I am attacking the Big Three relentlessly throughout this book, so let me state here that I am as susceptible to their appeal as is everyone else, and that I need to work as hard as most people in the struggle for moderation. But the focus of this book is not about us as adults; it's the role that the Big Three play in our children's diets.

Even if he or she is very healthy and maintains an appropriate weight for his or her height and age, the typical American child is still eating too much of the Big Three. Aside from the obvious front-burner issue of weight and obesity, a second major cause of concern that this poses is the role that the Big Three play in a national diet that is lacking in key nutrients. When kids opt for and fill up on snacks, sweet juices, fast foods, and other high fat and sweetened foods that don't deliver a lot of nutrients, there is not a lot of room left in the diet or the stomach for better foods.

And there is another question in all of this that is addressed far too seldom and, I believe, can lead to eating problems throughout childhood and even into adulthood. What does an overabundance in consumption of the Big Three do to a child's sense of natural flavor and taste?

Does eating too much fat, sodium, and/or sugar impede the proper palate development of a child and prevent him from learning to eat, appreciate, and prefer a broader range of foods? Yes, unequivocally. The "filler flavors" of the Big Three influence kids' palates to such a degree that the more diverse but often sub-tler flavors of foods that do not contain these properties cannot be enjoyed. Fat and salt are learned preferences, and the more that we are exposed to them, the more we crave them. Sweetness is more of an innate preference, but the human predilection for it is exacerbated by overexposure. Serve too much of any of the Big Three, and, eventually, acceptance or preference for other flavors will wilt.

When there is a preponderance of any one of the Big Three in a food, the flavor imparted by the added fat, sodium, or sugar has the unfortunate consequence of dominating the whole taste of the dish. That is why most fried foods, be they French fries, fried seafood, or fried chicken nuggets, taste a lot alike. You're not tast-ing the potato or the shrimp as much as you're tasting the oil used for frying. This is also true for soft drinks; of course you can tell a dark cola from other sodas, but they all taste similarly sweet. And it is the sweetness that lingers and defines what flavor there is in the beverage. Given that children are eating and drinking so many Big Three–laden products, there is not enough variety in the typical young child's diet to expose him to a wide range of food textures and flavors.

To say that this is a problem for all young children is a gener-alization and perhaps an overstatement, as of course there are many parents and caregivers who work very hard to monitor the foods that their charges are exposed to, trying as best as they can to steer youngsters toward healthful things. What concerns me most as a food professional and parent of two young children, however, is the proliferation of "kiddie foods" that provide *only* these elements—fat, sodium, and sugar—relying blatantly and exclusively on them to provide any "flavor" that the product has at all. Parents who want their kids to eat other things face a con-stant struggle against advertisers, many food companies, and even their own parent peers.

But That's What Kids Want to Eat, Right?

"Ha! Are you kidding? Let my kids choose their own meals,
completely? They wouldn't eat anything but hot dogs,
pretzels and dip, and cookies."
Dave, father of a six-year-old and a four-year-old,
when asked if a particular parenting approach
would work for his family

It might seem that this interest in children and what they eat is just another effect of the overall obsession with kids that seems to permeate American society. After all, children are groomed for the Ivy League or Major League Baseball or the role of Miss America before they set foot in elementary school. The level of obsession may be new, but the interest in kids and what they eat has been around for a long time, as evidenced by one of the first and most interesting detailed scientific studies ever done on the topic.

In 1939, pediatrician Clara Davis made a report at the annual meeting of the Canadian Medical Association that rocked conventional wisdom on the subject of kids and eating, and laid the foundation for a line of thinking to which many still subscribe today. In an era obviously very unlike our modern-day world, Davis was able to establish what amounted to an eating-observation lab that consisted of 15 children who lived in an orphanage. For over four years, every morsel of food or drop of a beverage consumed by these children was recorded, and height, weight, and blood levels were regularly monitored as well. This produced more than 36,000 individual data entries, long before there were Excel spreadsheets to record them.

The point? Dr. Davis wanted to see what children would choose to eat if they were left completely to their own devices, with no adult intervention or guidance at all. So these 15 kids were allowed to eat exactly what they wanted to eat, in whatever quantity appealed to them, for the entire four years. There were some limitations; notably, the children had just 33 individual food items to choose from, and all of the items were relatively nutritious. This meant that it would have been hard for any of them to consume a diet that was completely deficient nutritionally. (Davis was asked about that at the time and said that she wanted to do a follow-up study involving less nutritious processed foods, but that her funding ran out during the Great Depression.) And it turned out that all of the kids did, indeed, choose basically well-balanced diets, all on their own.

Despite some flaws in the research, what Davis found tells us a lot about kids' natural likes and dislikes regarding food. Most notably, none of the young children had the same diet on any given day, week, or month. "Every diet differed from every other diet, 15 different patterns of taste being presented, and not one diet was the predominantly cereal-and-milk diet, with smaller supplements of fruit, eggs, and meat, that is commonly thought proper," she reported.[4] This shocked physicians and nutritional experts of the day, who were used to prescribing very regimented, detailed eating plans for young kids. Davis was the first to declare that "children's bodies instinctively knew best," giving parents license to relax a bit. Dr. Benjamin Spock, the world's most famous pediatrician, became a champion of this attitude seven years later in the 1946 launch of his classic book *Baby and Child Care*,

"(Mothers) can trust an unspoiled child's appetite to choose a wholesome diet if she serves him a reasonable variety and balance of those natural and unrefined foods which he himself enjoys eating at present. Even more importantly, it means that she doesn't have to worry when he develops a temporary dislike of a vegetable."[5]

Dr. Davis's and Dr. Spock's comments apply, obviously, to young children who are still learning about new foods and teaching themselves how to eat. I doubt that either of them would advocate this concept in the case of older kids, and young teens, especially, allowing them to pick and choose their foods at will all of the time, and maintaining that a persistent avoidance of vegetables is nothing to worry about. Most important, we have to remember that these pediatricians practiced in an era before it was possible (and so very profitable) for food corporations and the media to target children as a segmented consumer group: advertise directly to them, design programming especially for them, and create food products just for undeveloped little taste buds.

Oh, for a simpler time.

What Makes It Harder Today

"The reality is, the marketing is in place. You can't beat that.
That's a very strong, powerful tool and they're being bombarded every
day. My daughter knew McDonald's name before she ever went there.
I don't know if you can beat it, but you can limit it."
Chef Steve Chiappetti of Viand Restaurant, Chicago,
father of a six-year-old and a three-year-old

Suppose you came home from work or running errands one day and discovered in your home a person whom you did not know, speaking in an animated and engaging voice to your young child. This person was showing your child all sorts of colorful packages of cereals, Popsicles, string cheeses, juices, and more, trying to persuade him or her to try a new flavor or "ask mom to serve you this for breakfast." You'd flip out, right?

And yet that's very close to what happens in virtually every American home, day after day, with kids' exposure to television advertising, says Dr. Jerome L. Singer, director of the Yale University

Television Research and Consultation Center. Other children or child-friendly adults, cartoon characters, animals, animated figures, or some such, "visit" your kids all the time, in the form of the thousands of exposures to advertisements for food products that children are bombarded with each year.

The average child watches about four hours of TV per day, says the American Academy of Pediatrics, and, in children's programming, sees over ten commercials for food products each hour. Almost 80% of the food products advertised are either high-sugar foods, such as candy, kids' cereals, and soft drinks, or convenience snack foods and fast foods.[6] And if the sheer volume of exposure to these so-called treats is not bad enough, remember this: until kids reach the age of about six, they can't distinguish commercials from regular programming. So a dancing Pop-Tart or a warrior candy bar in an advertisement is just as real to them as is a cartoon character on a program, or the actors on Blue's Clues, or the Wiggles. The "buy me" message, to kids, is part of the storyline.

And this is just television. Remember that these marketing whizzes out of the best MBA schools have also figured out a multitude of other ways to promote their products to your kids: interactive Web sites, programs conducted with reputable academic companies, coupon offers, character tie-ins, school and team sponsorships, promotional giveaways, and more. They even know what colors and type of packaging appeals most to kids, at every age level. It's depressing to realize, but I sometimes think they know more about my own kids' likes and dislikes than I do. Forty thousand times each year—that's over 100 times a day—the average child receives some sort of commercial product advertisement.[7]

This boom in media saturation dovetails nicely with a corresponding rise in the introduction of children's food products, which are coming out at a pace we've never seen before. U.S. food companies have introduced over 600 new children's food products since 1994; half of them candies or chewing gums, and a quarter more are other types of sweets or salty snacks.[8] Whether or not *you* would want to eat these particular new products is not relevant. Research and development teams at every many food corporations are hard at work, creating new foods just for little consumers. Marketing and advertising types then come up with packaging, advertisements, and all the bells and whistles, designed just for them. And we, as parents who may want to instill different "food values" in our kids, are left fighting not only an abundance issue, as a flood of these new kids products hits the store shelves each year, but also the incessant promotion of these products by manufacturers insistent upon creating demand.

One of my favorite authors is David Kamp, a contributing editor to *Vanity Fair* and *GQ* magazines, who is also the father of two. His 2007 book, *The United States of Arugula: How We Became a Gourmet Nation*, is an eminent contribution to literature on American culinary history, as well as a fascinating read. "When I was growing up, 'kids' food' meant a Popsicle from the Good Humor ice cream truck, not an entire industry devoted to churning out new products," said this member of Generation X. "Breakfast was the only meal of the day where there was any delineation between what the kids ate and what our parents ate," he added, referring to such perennial kids' favorites as Frosted Flakes and Fruit Loops.

Yes, food options, not to mention the promotion of them, for children born at the dawn of the twenty-first century are quite different from what they were in the pre-TV days of 1939, when Dr. Clara Davis presented her research, or 1946, when Dr. Spock first came onto the scene, or even when you and I were growing up. In past eras, we could assume that kids would be eating the same things that the adults around them ate, in lesser quantities and perhaps not all at once, but eventually, naturally, evolving in this direction. Now, if you want your kids to grow up with an interest in food, a knowledge of skills for healthful eating, and an appreciation of flavors, you're really taking your chances if you let go of all concern about what they eat as youngsters.

Something else that's different for our kids today: the concept of certain foods as "treats" is almost completely gone. A stop at an ice cream parlor after a big outing, special candies at birthday parties, holiday goodies from year to year—stop and think about your childhood memories and the role that foods played in some of them. Now look at your kid's lives and compare how these "treats" have become such an everyday occurrence, something so expected and ubiquitous and handed out on every occasion, that they have lost any semblance of distinction.

"Oh, this is a special treat," we tell ourselves as justification for doling out goodies to our kids. But look at it as part of the big picture of the overall diet, and it's very likely that it's just more of the same thing that is eaten every other day. Processed sugar or fat or sodium in another form, perhaps, but in reality, just more of the same.

One obvious effect of a transformation of treats into everyday fare is an increase in the amount of high calorie, low nutrient foods that make up children's everyday diets. And as with many things that become too familiar in our lives, what once was viewed as exceptional is now just "ordinary."

America vs. the World: Are Our Kids Behind in the Flavor Game?

"In this country, we cater so much to kids when it comes to food. I have friends who put four or five things out before they find something their children will eat. In other countries, like where I'm from [Lebanon], kids don't have a choice. Now, I just give my daughter whatever I'm eating, and she loves it."
Grace, mother of a two-year-old and a five-month-old

One of my favorite memories of our son Willie's babyhood came when he was about nine months old, during a family vacation to Playa del Carmen, Mexico. Willie happily gobbled up the local fruits, such as mangoes and plantains, as well as dishes such as guacamole and black beans that we found in the restaurants. This was one of those times when we also wanted to have commercial baby foods on hand, however, so I went to a local grocery store to see what was available.

It was interesting to scan the shelves and learn that, according to Gerber at least, infants in Mexico are interested in different foods than are infants in America. You will find in Mexican stores a whole range of baby food products that reflect the local cuisine: pureed mangoes, black beans and rice, strained plantains, mixed papaya and guava, chayotes. These are all packaged in the same familiar jars and plastic packets with the Gerber baby on the front that you find here in the United States. But read the labels and the lists of products offered around the world, and you may begin to feel really sorry for American babies. Clearly, the assumption about our kids' preferred foods and eating patterns is different from that of children in other countries. A call to Gerber confirms this. "When possible, our products are localized to adapt to the cuisine of the culture," a representative told me.

Take a look at some of the baby foods that Gerber offers around the world, but not in the United States:

♦ *Mexico:*
Guava, Papaya and Guava, Green Beans and Ham, Herbed Salmon, Chayotes, Plantains

♦ *Russia:*
Broccoli, Pumpkin, Potato, Cauliflower, Lamb

♦ *Venezuela:*
Guava, Mango, Plum, Papaya

♦ *Poland:*
Raspberries, Broccoli, Fish

A Korean baby food company has dishes for nine-month-olds that are flavored with seaweed; for year-old babies, they offer radish roots and soft tofu.

I point this out not to bemoan a shortage in varietals of commercial baby foods in this country, but rather as validation that a leading company in a major food industry has recognized that babies growing up in other parts of the world are expected to adapt their palates to their regional cuisines. Parents elsewhere are eating different things, and they want their children to eat those things. And as the kids progress to table foods, these infants will learn to enjoy their native dishes, which are often spicier, richer, fresher, and more flavorful than what young American children typically eat.

Why have we in this country come to assume that babies and young children should and will only eat certain "kid-oriented" foods? The bland baby cereals, the sweet beverages and fruits (as opposed to vegetables), the salty, and the fried?

In researching this book, I sought input from non-American-born parents of young children, as well as American parents raising their kids in other countries, asking them to compare the norm in infant feeding in the United States to their homeland or country of residence. What surprised me most was not the answers I received, but the intensity with which the issue was discussed. Across the board, parents from other countries stressed that in their home nations, mothers and fathers generally feed their children "homemade foods," "real foods," and "adult foods" much more often and at younger ages than we typically do in this country. Cost was sometimes mentioned as the major reason that this is the case, as commercial baby foods are even more expensive in some other countries than they are in the United States. But also discussed were more personal points: "Babies and young children are seen as part of the family, and that includes what they eat." "We take a lot of pride in our cooking and cuisine and can't imagine feeding our children anything else." Or, my personal favorite: "Why *wouldn't* they eat what we eat?"

Grace was born in Lebanon, moved to the United States as a young child, and grew up in her family's Lebanese restaurant business. She is now the mother of a two-year-old daughter and an infant son. Her little girl loves traditional Middle Eastern dishes such as kibbeh, hummus, kebobs, and falafels. "Infants in Lebanon are exposed to solid foods earlier than they traditionally are here, and they also try a lot of new foods earlier," Grace said. As a result of raising her own children this way, "My daughter eats exactly what I'm eating. She never questions what is put before her; that's the meal."

A lot of American kids do visit Lebanese Taverna, Grace's family's restaurant, and are often surprised to find out how much they like the intense spices of the foods. "If they will just try a different cuisine, most kids will love it, because the food really is very, very good. Lebanese food has an emphasis on intense flavorings. It's very different from traditional American food, but that can be a good thing if kids and their parents can get over their fear of trying it.

"We offer foods that may look and sound a little familiar to American kids, but are distinctly Middle Eastern in substance," she continued. "We have a Middle Eastern–style pizza that is made in a wood-burning oven, as well as things like shrimp kebobs and a kastaburger that is made of ground beef and spices and served on a pita bread. There is a macaroni bel haleg that is Lebanese pasta with a béchamel sauce. It's essentially pasta and a milk sauce. What child wouldn't like that?"

Missionaries and teachers in Ethiopia, Mike and Janelle moved to a rural area there when their now four-year-old daughter Carolee was just a year old. "She didn't eat packaged baby or toddler foods because there were none," Mike told me. "We just gave her what-ever was available to us, which was mainly things like root crops, lots of beans, and vegetables."

Mike added that children in Ethiopia typically begin eating native foods at around age two-and-a-half, perhaps prepared with a bit less spice than adult fare until they are about five.

When Mike and Janelle recently moved back to the United States, they noticed that Carolee was much less of a picky eater than many of the kids here. "She still loves to eat all vegetables, cooked and uncooked, and snacks on things like nuts, seeds, fruits, and whole grains," Mike told me. "Her transition back to eating in America was mostly smooth, although she was over-whelmed at first by all of the variety in food choices and brands that were thrust upon her at once. The biggest difference between Carolee and most other kids her age here is that she won't eat breaded and fried foods. She doesn't like them at all."

I heard similar stories from other parts of the world, especially Europe. There is France, of course, where children in all of the 270 public daycare centers in Paris receive a fresh meal prepared by a chef each day. These mostly organic dishes might include pasta salad with decorative tomato skin flower petals, cauliflower au gratin, and braised lamb in fresh rosemary, according to a National Public Radio report. "Presentation is very important," one of the chefs said. "Before tasting, you look. So when you see something nice, you want to eat it."

"These lunches help children develop the potential to enjoy a proper sit-down meal with an appetizer, main plate, cheese, and a dessert, while taking their time in a convivial atmosphere," adds a dietitian for the Paris daycare system. And all at a cost of about $2 per meal per child.

My friend Maria is from Seville, Spain, the mother of a five-year-old boy and the wife of an American Midwesterner, who had to get used to the idea of feeding him on a Spanish schedule.

"In Spain, kids eat out at restaurants late at night all the time," Maria said. "It's nothing for young children to be in restaurants having dinner at ten o'clock at night." As soon as her young son started eating table foods, Maria started him on a Spanish eating schedule: an early morning piece of fruit, followed by a snack, such as a small serving of yogurt, around 11:00 a.m. They then have a big lunch, such as a salad and fish with fruit for dessert, around 2:00 in the afternoon. Late afternoon is time for milk and a small sandwich, followed by a dinner of chicken or something similar or an omelet late at night.

My friend Sabrina grew up in Washington, D.C., and now lives in Southern Italy with her husband and two young children. When her baby daughter started on infant cereals, she was advised to mix them with vegetable broth made with carrots, potatoes, and zucchini, rather than water, as is typical in the United States. A simple introduction to flavor, at a very early age! And, Sabrina adds, "At first Giada didn't like the rice cereals, so our pediatrician recommended adding a little bit of grated Parmigiano cheese." How Italian is that?

And Irina, from Russia, told me that mothers there almost always prepare fruits and vegetables at home for their infants and children, and that some of the American commercial baby foods sold there seem odd, because they are for foods that are not native to the country. "Green beans and sweet potatoes aren't grown in Russia, and these items as prepared baby foods are very expensive," she said. "So people just cook the things from their own gardens for their babies, like potatoes, carrots, beets, zucchini, turnips, apples, pears, and plums." Irina added that often Russian babies are fed homemade soups, which are very thick and more like our stews. Another old Russian tradition that is still followed in many places is giving very young babies, around three or four months old, sour milk products, such as cottage cheese and sour cream.

Monica Bhide, born in Delhi and reared in Bahrain, is now a cooking teacher and cookbook author, and the mother of two sons, aged eight years and fifteen months. She moved to the United States when she was 21, having never had a McDonald's hamburger, but growing up fascinated by American food culture after watching television programs such as "The Cosby Show." "They would eat peanut butter and jelly sandwiches, and I would ask my dad: How can they puree peanuts? What are they thinking?" Monica said. "He said, 'Well, you eat almond butter; it's the same idea.'"

She is raising her sons with an interest in food from her international perspective. "Because of my profession, I'm constantly testing new recipes at home—everything from Thai and Malaysian to Indian to typical American dishes. I think that sort of encourages my boys to not be afraid of different foods," Monica says. "Even as young as three, my boys would go to the grocery store and be able to pick up ginger or garlic, or tell cilantro from the herbs. They'd take it out of the cart and go, 'Eggplant, potato, tomato . . .'."

When Monica and her husband take their kids to India, they adapt immediately to the food there. "I think my mom tends to cook a little bit spicier so they found food a little bit hot," she said. "They found some of the fruits fascinating. They loved getting coconut water out on the street—that was a big thing.

"And the McDonald's in India serves really different food, things like vegetarian burgers with spicy chutney, or a paneer roll. Instead of giving away toys like they do here, they give away things like books on cricket."

Japanese-American Chieko and her husband live in Washington, D.C., with their four-year-old son Chase and Chieko's Japanese mother. The confluence of cultures has been interesting to them, especially as they watch their young son learn to eat new foods. Although he is being raised speaking Japanese at home and with the strong influence of his mother's heritage, Chieko says that Chase is a pickier eater and eats a less varied diet than do children in Japan, simply because he is living in the United States. "In Japan, the schools really emphasize variety and nutrition in kids' lunches, even if they are brought from home," Chieko told me. "There is an established, minimum number of ingredients that should be found in the lunchbox, and an emphasis on a variety of colors in food." Clean plates are also important in Japanese schools, as children are taught that an uneaten lunch would be disrespectful to their mother, whose hard work would have gone to waste.

"Mothers (in Japan) spend a lot of time and energy planning meals, so if Japanese moms saw the Lunchables that are for sale in grocery stores here, they would faint from shock," she added.

Little Chase has the advantage of having his grandmother living with him as well, so he gets the full benefit of Japanese influence in his diet. "One thing my mother and I have noticed with Americans is that there is very little concept of enjoying 'hot things hot and cold things cold.' Chieko says that her mother's biggest pet peeve is when things that are supposed to be served hot, soup for example, are allowed to sit on the table to cool because the person being served doesn't like hot things. "Imagine her surprise when we had a few people with young children over for a pizza-making party one day," Chieko said. "The pizza was warm, not piping hot, actually at the perfect temperature. One father opened the freezer door and put a slice of pizza inside because he was afraid to give hot food to his three-year-old." Chase handles hot foods well now, she says, because of their insistence that everything be served to him at the appropriate temperature.

"The other thing that I think is important in Japanese culture but missing in America, especially when it comes to kids, is the concept of 'presentation' of foods," Chieko continued, noting that in Japan, how food looks is as important as how it tastes. "We went to a pancake place for breakfast one morning with some other families, and one of the little boys, who was about five years old, was away from the table when his pancake order arrived. My mother was shocked that his mother proceeded to cut up the pancakes before he got there into child-size bites, without giving him a chance to see what the whole dish looked like. All he saw when he got to the table was a mess of pieces of food. I know that parents here do that a lot. We certainly cut up Chase's food for him, but only a few bites at a time, so that his plate looks as much as possible like the adult plates."

I love that. Sure, it's probably a little more work for parents, but what a nice way to instill respect for the food and the work that went into preparing it. To children, it sends the subtle message: Stop before you dig in. Think about what you're eating and appreciate it, rather than just look at food as something to fill a hunger void. And taking the time to create a nice presentation on the plate may have the added positive effect of teaching your child something about proper portion sizes, a concept that many adults seem to have lost track of.

After hearing stories like this from so many parents about how babies and young children around the world eat, I actually started to feel a little sorry for American kids! Here we are with all this abundance and quantity of food products, and yet very little thought is given to how food actually tastes to them. Our mindset is more along the lines of bland foods for infants, starting with rice cereals and such, leading to first foods that still have little in the way of seasoning. In our care to ensure that each new food is introduced properly, allowing time to register any sensitivities and allergies, we seem to go on caution overload and forget that flavor is also something that we need to teach children about their food, along with feeding skills, portion control, and nutrition.

In the words of Chef Marc Murphy of New York's Landmarc Restaurant, "As I always say to people who tell me that their kids don't eat spicy things: 'What do you think kids in Mexico eat? Not eat jalapeños?' Or they'll say their kids don't eat sushi; do you think in Japan the children don't eat sushi? It's ludicrous!"

All of these conversations inspired me to contact Dr. Nancy Butte, a professor of pediatrics at Baylor College of Medicine and a researcher at the school's Children's Nutrition Research Center. Dr. Butte is a leader in the field of childhood obesity, looking for its causes in both environmental and genetic issues. She has compared childhood feeding traditions across various cultures, studying the ways that we introduce solids and table foods to infants and toddlers. In a 2006 interview with *Time* magazine, Dr. Butte is quoted as saying, "There is no good reason to feed babies bland food. It's culturally determined, not scientifically based." I asked her about these conflicting norms in feeding young children.

"In other countries, babies start on various gruels, soups, porridges, and purees, similar to our rice and other cereals. From there, teaching young infants to eat solid foods is a culturally specific progression," Dr. Butte told me. "Manufacturers in the United States sell baby foods based on mothers' expectations and preferences; for example, stage one foods are usually fruit and stage threes might have some meat. But the order in which foods are introduced really doesn't seem to matter, so long as they are introduced one at a time to watch for adverse reactions. Pureed meats make a good first food, along with cereals, because they provide the nutrient iron, which begins to diminish in breast milk after about six months of lactation."

"Between twelve and twenty-four months, young toddlers should be transitioning onto the family diet. And unfortunately, that's when food choices may not be optimal for young American children."

What I've Learned

— On the basis of individual, day-by-day situations, it may appear that young children's diets aren't that bad, or at least no worse than those of the rest of us. You see a kid eating a children's cereal, drinking juice from a box, or ordering a grilled cheese sandwich at a nice Italian restaurant and you think, "Oh, well, that's what kids do." But then you realize that these aren't isolated incidents; it's what so many kids do all of the time, and worse, it's all they know in the way of food-related experiences.

— The number one reason that so many kids eat this way is that they are not only allowed to, but they are encouraged to. It's expected; it's easy.

— At some point, most parents get a bit desperate when they realize what they have wrought. The five- or six-year-old who refuses to eat vegetables and demonstrates other picky eater qualities is difficult not only to live with, but to change. And so the typical concerned parent tries to work with the existing situation by employing creative ways to get nutrients into the kid, without actually forcing a confrontation. From this, elaborate schemes, such as baking pureed cauliflower into cakes, are born.

— Even if you are vigilant about your child's eating habits from an early age, even if you get off to a great start and produce a pint-sized foodie, even if you do everything "right," you will still be amazed and probably caught off guard by the strength of the advertising and promotional might of many food companies and the power and influence that these will eventually hold over your children and his or her peers.

— In all likelihood, your young child's contemporaries living in many foreign lands may be eating better than your child is—a more varied diet, a healthier diet, a tastier diet. While they may not have as much food or nearly as many different brands to choose from, chances are they are being fed less-processed, healthier foods from a younger age. There are many reasons for this, chief among them the fact that non-American parents are not as exposed to, nor captivated and influenced by, messages from the commercial formula and baby food industries as we are.

CHAPTER 3

⌘

You Can't Start Too Soon

"I was not raised as an adventurous eater. I'm still often flummoxed by what to order in fancy restaurants. I think I'm like a lot of other people. I never learned to use chopsticks. I've never had Ethiopian or Korean food. Now my dessert is always Lipitor."
NBC *Nightly News* anchor Brian Williams,
speaking to *Parade* magazine, November 16, 2008

L ooking back on my children's launch into the food world, I can see that much of the groundwork was laid before they ever started to eat real food and, on some points, before they were born. You are ahead of the game if you start with parents who are committed to the same goal and put it into practice in their own lives, before little ones even enter the picture.

My husband Paul grew up on a farm in south-central Pennsyl-vania and started eating a bounty of local fruits and vegetables at a very young age. He has fond memories of trips to the market to help sell home-grown produce with his grandparents. Paul even ties this early love of farming and appreciation for locally based food to his adult profession. He still talks with enthusiasm about a first trip to Europe almost thirty years ago, where he sampled local wines served with regional cuisine. That first experience of eating in this typically European style set him on the path to a career in the wine retail industry.

My own interest in food had a more prosaic beginning. I sort of wandered into the culinary world by way of business interests. I spent many years developing marketing and communications skills in the food industry while working at a large public rela-tions agency. It was there, working with top chefs, world-class restaurants, cooking schools, and international food companies, that I began to appreciate the value and enjoyment that food can bring. I began immersing myself in culinary matters by taking cooking classes, reading cookbooks and cooking publications, and becoming a bit of a chef-and-restaurant groupie. My own palate has developed and evolved along the way, which is why I feel so strongly that children's taste preferences can also be trained and influenced. Just enjoying what you eat is the best first step.

I admit, though, that I did not picture an easy transition from cooking and dining as a couple, to feeding young children and eating as a family, at least not at first. One night when I was preg-nant with Willie, Paul and I were talking about the changes that we had ahead of us. "I guess we won't be cooking a lot of big din-ners for awhile," I said, "and how are we ever going to eat out? What will the baby eat?"

"The baby will eat what we eat," he replied matter-of-factly, and that statement must have made quite an impression on me, because I remember it very well to this day. "Oh, right. Of course. You don't *have* to give them jarred baby food!"

It Starts with an Attitude

"My husband and I, and just about everyone in our extended families, love food. We're OK cooks, not the best, but we all enjoy trying new things both at home and at restaurants. I love walking through the produce aisle or a farmer's market and seeing all of the beautiful foods. A good meal makes my day!"
Anna, mother of a four-year-old

(Sigh) "I guess I have to go to the grocery store. Again."
Me, too often

(Which of these people would you rather spend time with?!)

Think about your own relationship with food. Do you "hate" to cook or grocery shop, and not mind telling anyone so? Do you gravitate to the same restaurants, the same three or four quick dinner recipes, the same brand of cereal or snack food, "the usual" when you eat out? There's nothing wrong with having favorites, of course, but there is a fine line between being in a comfortable routine and being in a real rut. Branching out and trying new things in the kitchen or at a restaurant can be daunting and maybe even disappointing. Many people don't want to take any chances. Food is expensive; what if I ruin a challenging recipe? What if a new restaurant lets me down, or if I try a different menu item and I don't like it as much as what I regularly order? Or, probably most common, I'm in a hurry, dealing with a lot of issues, and need some level of predictability in my day. Meals can provide that. There's a lot to be said for opting for the easy choice when we are overwhelmed.

It's also easy to let thoughts about food variety and nutrition slip when it's just you, or just the two of you. You work out, you had a fruit salad on Tuesday, you skip lunch most days to cut down on calories; of course you're taking care of yourself. What difference does it make if "dinner," such as it is, is in reality more like a sandwich in front of the television at midnight or a bowl of cold cereal after a long day?

It might not make much difference in your life, but when you're trying to influence a young child, who has neither the knowledge base from which to make taste and flavor comparisons nor the judgment to decide for himself what he should eat, it becomes an important matter. It's up to us as parents to teach those skills. And like many areas of parenting, what you do and what you say can really make an impact.

How often do you hear adults talking about their own dietary limitations, foods they don't like or even "hate," and their disdain for cooking? "My husband is a meat and potatoes guy; he would never eat that," is a phrase I hear often from women. "If the Smiths are coming over, we'd better just order pizza; there are too many things they won't eat." Or, "I'm on a diet and I can't be bad again today and have a dessert." If young children are in the house, you can bet that they pick up on these statements and incorporate them into their own thinking. Even worse is when adults make definitive comments about not liking entire categories of food. Personal preferences and negative generalizations become the subject of too much conversation, as in: "I don't eat spicy foods," "He doesn't eat seafood," "Uncle Mike doesn't like vegetables," "I tried that once and didn't like it." And on and on.

Remember that all of this chatter is heard and absorbed by little ears and gives kids an as-yet undeserved license to judge foods. So if you find that you or your spouse are falling into these habits, be aware and make a commitment to make only positive comments about food when children are around. Like or dislike something all you want; just don't pass your personal sentiments about these issues on to your kids.

I was reminded of how easy it is to slip up on this when I was in the car one day with Willie, and we drove past a favorite restaurant. To my surprise, it had a big "Closed Permanently" sign on the door, and the windows were shuttered. "What happened?" Willie asked. "I don't know," I said. "I guess the chef just got tired of cooking." "Like you are tired of cooking for us boys?" he asked. I paused, remembering the grumbling I had been doing of late about another meal to prepare, another trip to the grocery store.

If attitude adjustments among parents or other adults who are in frequent contact with the child are in order, now is the time to make those changes. For example, while husband Paul will admit that he can be a real food snob, refusing to eat produce before or after its peak or pointing out when certain dishes are over- or under-salted, he does adhere to a basic guideline that we established when Willie entered the picture. We try very hard never to state blanket dislike or criticism of a particular food in front of him, even if it is something that we don't particularly enjoy eating. And we try to reinforce the lessons of variety and adventure in eating by choosing new restaurants, new foods, and new recipes whenever possible. If something flops, so be it; *"Well, at least we tried!"* is the motto.

Live a Little!

"So when I became governor, I fired the personal chef, much to my kids' dismay. I said, 'Mac and cheese is fine for them.'"
Former Alaska governor and 2008 vice-presidential candidate
Sarah Palin, on the campaign stump

"Sometimes they look at things and say, 'It's green.' (The White House chefs) have done a great job in meeting the taste needs of a seven- and ten-year-old. They make mean French fries, waffles, and grits."
First Lady Michelle Obama, shortly after moving
into the White House

Hemant Singh is a charming waiter at the trendy Bluepointe restaurant in Atlanta, where Chef Doug Turbush turns out a fantastic array of sushi and contemporary Asian-American dishes. With sleek décor and a crowded sushi bar scene, Bluepointe is not the type of restaurant that you'd expect would draw a lot of kids. Still, Singh says that every few days, he does have a table that includes young children. "And I spend a lot of time encouraging the children or their parents to order an interesting dish," said Singh. "Even in a place like this, where we offer amazing seafood and meat dishes paired with interesting vegetables and flavorful Asian sauces, the typical default order for children is still pasta or chicken fingers.

"But a lot of adults are just as bad," Singh continues. "I don't understand why more people don't use dining-out experiences to try something new, especially when there is a top chef cooking for you."

Published research on children's food acceptance patterns documents the important role that parents' attitudes about food plays in setting the stage for Junior to develop a broad palate. A 1996 study of 57 families in two Swedish towns examined children's reasons for liking or disliking certain foods, as well as the reasons for rejection of foods served in the family. Through questionnaires and interviews on food preferences, they found that the higher the "Picky Eater" rating of the mothers and their children, the lower the range of variety of foods served in the home.[9] And a 1998 University of Tennessee study had similar findings when it examined the food preferences of 118 toddlers, ages 28 months to three years old. All of these children's parents or adult caregivers were asked to fill out a questionnaire about their own personal likes and dislikes concerning food. They then filled out an identical form on behalf of their youngsters. In these questionnaires, 196 commonly eaten foods were listed, and everyone was asked to rate it as a "like," "dislike," "never offered," or "never tasted."

No surprise: there was a strong correlation (more than 80%) of food preferences between the children and their parents. But again, here's that important point: the researchers also found a significant similarity between foods never offered to the child and the mothers' dislikes. Of all the 196 foods named, 31 were not eaten by a majority of the toddlers because they had never been offered to them. That list included such wonderful possibilities as lamb chops, avocado, winter squash, beets, and pork chow mein.[10] "Parents and caregivers should not prejudge or stereotype foods they 'think' the child will not like and eat; rather, they should expose them to a wide variety of foods," the study concluded. What better way to do that than to start now, eating a broader variety of foods yourself, and perhaps even making a conscious attempt to retry some foods that you haven't eaten in a long time because you're sure you don't like them?

These same Tennessee researchers (Betty Ruth Carruth, PhD, RD, and Jean Skinner, PhD, RD) went on to conduct many other studies on children's eating habits during their careers in academia. In another well-publicized trial, their research followed 70 mother–child pairs, from the time the children were infants until they were eight years old. Carruth and Skinner confirmed that mothers' and children's food preferences were significantly related, again primarily because foods disliked by mothers tended not to be offered to the kids. "Mothers influence children via their own preferences," the authors wrote. "It is unlikely that children will be accepting of unfamiliar foods if the parents exhibit (fear of new food) traits."[11]

"It is worthwhile to encourage parents to offer their children as wide a variety of foods as possible, including foods that the parents themselves dislike. Denying young children the opportunity to taste a wide variety of foods may limit their range of acceptable foods as they mature," the Carruth and Skinner report concluded.

For parents or parents-to-be, expanding their own food repertoire, even just a little, is a crucial first step. "About 20% of people eat a diet composed entirely of just 10 or fewer foods," reports *Woman's Day* magazine. Don't let that be you! Now you have a perfect excuse for you, your spouse, family members, and other adults who will eventually influence your child to branch out a little bit! Try something different *today* when making your own food choices. Sample that new piece of produce you see at the grocery store, prepare a recipe from a friend's cookbook, try the chef's special on a menu, or even try that strange-looking dish that your mother-in-law insists on bringing to every family function. And if you're someone who confuses the food guide pyramid with the Golden Arches, this is as good a time as any to pay more attention to nutrition aspects of your diet. Make a conscious effort to be more curious and adventuresome when it comes to food. You get full points just for trying, and who knows—you might find something new that you really like.

Mom-to-Be: You (and Your Child) Are What You Eat

"Pop-Tarts, which I've never eaten before in my life. Pomegranate juice with club soda. Chocolate dipped in almond butter. You name it, if it was weird, I had a craving for it when I was pregnant."
Sarah, mom to a now four-month-old

The test says yes, the doctor confirms it, and here you are: stunned, elated, anxious, and so much more, all at the same time. You're pregnant! And suddenly, the phrase "you are what you eat" takes on a whole new meaning.

Whether you're ravenously hungry, can't keep a bite of food down for days at a time, or haven't noticed any real changes in your food consumption yet, you will, at some point, come to realize the importance of food issues during pregnancy. The list of "don'ts"—raw seafood, unpasteurized cheeses and juices, swordfish and other fish that accumulate mercury, alcoholic beverages—is there, as is the list of "do's"—fruits and vegetables, especially, along with milk, proteins, and other elements of a healthful diet. Is pregnancy a time to eat more or less? Cravings may be huge or nonexistent, and do they mean anything? (An old wives' tale is that sour or salty means it's a boy, while sweets predict a girl. That was certainly true in my case, when I, a bona fide chocoholic, didn't care for the stuff and instead gorged on oranges and various cheeses during both of my pregnancies.) Welcome to the nine (fleeting) months that you are truly "eating for two (or more)"!

You can get plenty of nutrition advice from your health practitioner, by talking to experienced moms, or by reading some of the many books and articles available on the subject of what to eat and what to avoid eating while pregnant. But in the spirit of this book and in the interest of getting a little food lover off to a good start, I'll stick to looking at these questions from another point of view: does what an expectant mother eats during pregnancy, and later if she's breastfeeding, affect the eventual palate development of the growing child?

I first became interested in this issue through the most unlikely of circumstances: during a conversation with Paul about his life growing up on a Pennsylvania farm, and hearing his stories of how his grandfather had to make valiant efforts to keep the cows on a certain side of the pasture. Why? "Because if they wandered into an area that had wild onions in the grass, their milk would stink and taste awful for days," he informed me, truly amazing this city girl. Well, gee, I remember thinking, if you can tell the difference with that small of a change in a cow's diet, what must that say about the milk that humans produce to feed their infants? Most of us have a much more varied diet than your average cow.

One of the most interesting places that I've come in contact with during my career in the food industry is the Monell Chemical Senses Center in Philadelphia. Founded in 1968 for the purpose of "advancing knowledge of the mechanisms and functions of the chemical senses, (such as) taste and smell," Monell today boasts over 100 scientists and technicians who study all aspects of these senses. Their work is supported by foundations and industry grants. Faculty member Julie Mennella, PhD, is known for her research work in the development of flavor preferences in humans, so she was just the person to take this question to. Mennella has published a multitude of papers and studies on the subject in numerous acclaimed scientific journals. She says that science shows that a mother's diet is the first stage in the long process of how humans learn about new dietary flavors.

One of her early studies (1995) looked at the effect of garlic consumption on expectant moms' amniotic fluid. Amniotic fluid, as you probably recall, surrounds, protects, and provides a source of nourishment to the growing baby. Samples of amniotic fluid were obtained from 10 pregnant women during their routine amniocentesis tests. Forty-five minutes prior to the screening, five of the women swallowed a capsule containing essence of garlic oil, while the other half ingested a placebo. Comparisons of the fluid from the two groups found that four of the five women who consumed garlic oil produced amniotic fluid with a stronger odor, "more like actual garlic."[12]

OK, so the amniotic fluid is affected by mom's diet. But does that translate to a direct effect on Baby, once he or she is born? Apparently so. In a study conducted about the same time in Ireland, researchers tested infants 20 hours after their births to determine their response to garlic. Babies whose mothers ate no garlic during their pregnancies showed an aversion to the odor, while those who had been exposed during their mothers' pregnancies showed no aversion.[13]

We also know that newborns can pick out the scent of their own amniotic fluid. French researchers observing three-day-old breastfed and bottle-fed infants found that they all turned their heads toward their own, familiar amniotic fluid, as opposed to another infant's fluid.[14] "Within days of birth, babies gravitate toward the odor of their own amniotic fluid, which suggests that prenatal sensory experiences can bias the newborn's behaviors and preferences," writes French researcher Benoist Schaal, who found similar results with newborns' familiarity with anise flavors consumed by their mothers.[15] Schaal's study also confirmed that babies born to moms who did not consume anise during their pregnancy likewise displayed aversion to that odor. Researchers go so far as to point to these "very early flavor experiences as the foundation for cultural and ethnic differences in cuisine."[16]

Mennella and her Monell colleagues conducted another fascinating experiment in which they were able to see—literally—the impact that a mom-to-be's food choices had on Baby, even months after birth, as the child was being breastfed and then learning to eat solid foods. Expectant women were asked to consume just over a cup of either carrot juice or water, four days a week for three weeks, either during the last months of their pregnancy or during the first two months that they were breastfeeding. Some months later, after the babies had started eating cereal but not much else, they were given carrot juice, mixed in with their cereal.

Researchers videotaped the babies during this particular eating session so that they could watch their little expressions and reactions as they were exposed to this new food. The results? The babies who had tasted carrots previously, through exposure from amniotic fluid or breast milk, made fewer "negative facial expressions" (anyone who has watched a baby eat knows what that means!) than did the babies whose mothers had had only water during the testing period. Those with previous experience were much more receptive initially to the taste of the carrots.[17] Mennella confirmed that the flavors of different foods enter the mother's milk at different rates, based on how fat-soluble they are, but they all eventually end up influencing the taste of the milk to some degree.

So evidence is in that flavor development and appreciation starts early—very early—in our lives. In fact, it appears that what we feed our infants and the flavors that we expose them to in their earliest days goes on to influence food acceptance patterns down the line, when they are toddlers and young children. But even if the results from these many existing studies don't apply in every case—well, hey, pregnant mom, why take the chance? We spend so much time and energy and thought taking care of ourselves and our bodies during this prenatal period in other ways, why not think about the impact of adding flavor to your child's life now? If expectant moms eat a wide flavor profile during pregnancy, apparently, it can only increase the odds that the child will enjoy eating a variety of foods a couple of years later.

From Day One: A Milk Diet

"I look at it this way: I don't give my two older kids processed, pack-aged, or canned foods. Why would I give this to a newborn?"
Anna, mom to a six-year-old, three-year-old, and two-month-old

"I was given formula. My mother drank formula when she was a baby.
I'm giving my daughter formula. We're all just fine."
Elizabeth, mom to a four-month-old

So much of pregnancy and childbirth is unpredictable, but of one thing you can be sure: soon after birth, assuming all goes well, of course, Baby will have her first "meal," and it will be some form of milk. And as you will quickly learn, whether you go breast or bottle to provide your baby that milk is a big decision, prime for more weigh-ins from outside sources.

Three out of four new mothers in this country—77%—now breastfeed their infants for at least a brief period of time, reports the Centers for Disease Control and Prevention. This is the highest breastfeeding rate in the United States in the last 20 years. This very good news is likely the result of ongoing educational campaigns designed to encourage more women to breastfeed. Healthy People 2010, for example, a federally funded prevention initiative to improve the health of all Americans, had set 75% of women as a target goal by 2010, and has programs in place to support these efforts. As of 2008, 42% of mothers were still breastfeeding when their children were six months old, and 21% were at one year. This is up substantially from 10 years earlier, in 1998, when only 29% of women were still breastfeeding at that important six-month mark.[18]

Here are two upfront statements about my views on this subject, as I don't want my opinion to cloud what can be a touchy subject. First, I am a very strong advocate of breastfeeding over formula feeding, based on the piles of scientific evidence that demonstrate that it is truly what is best for both the health of babies and their moms. Breastfeeding and formula feeding are not interchangeable; one is clearly superior to the other. Breast milk contains several hundred ingredients, all of them natural and many of them live antibodies that can never be reproduced in formula. A mother's milk changes and adapts to her growing baby's specific needs. The World Health Organization, the American Academy of Pediatrics, the American College of Obstetrics and Gynecology, and many other leading health groups are very clear about this: exclusive breastfeeding for the first six months of life is the optimal way to feed infants.

That said, I fully recognize that for whatever reason some—not many, but some—new mothers simply cannot nurse their babies and must rely on alternate feeding. Also, the many infants who are fortunate enough to be adopted into loving homes usually miss out on this benefit. But I also believe that the number of women who give birth and then truly cannot breastfeed is a very small percentage, and the great majority of women who formula-feed do so by choice. And while there might be perfectly valid reasons for this choice, I believe that we need to be more supportive, promotional, and encouraging of breastfeeding in this country than we currently are. More women need to be told of the benefits of breastfeeding more often, and need to be assisted with it when there are problems, and encouraged to keep it up for as long as possible. Quite frankly, the formula option is just made too easy in our culture.

In his acclaimed *Baby and Child Care*, the venerable pediatrician Benjamin Spock put it this way: "Why is it that throughout most of the world a mother's milk takes care of the baby for many months and that it's only in bottle-feeding countries like ours that the breast milk supply seems to fail so early in a majority of cases? . . . I think there is one main reason. The mother here who is trying to breast-feed, instead of feeling that she is doing the most natural thing in the world and assuming that she'll succeed like everyone else, feels that she's attempting to do the unusual, the difficult thing. Unless she has tremendous self-confidence she keeps wondering whether she won't fail."

"The way to make breast-feeding a success is to go on breast-feeding and keep away from formula," he adds.

"About 1% of new mothers truly cannot breastfeed their infants, due to a medical or physiological condition, such as a low milk supply," says Pat Shelly, a registered nurse and board-certified lactation consultant who directs the Breastfeeding Center of Washington, D.C. "In addition, another 1% of babies simply can't do it, for whatever physical reason. And beyond that, maybe 10 to 20% of women need assistance and intervention to make breastfeeding work." Shelly, who has taught classes and counseled thousands of women during her 12 years at the Center, adds that there may be some correlation between women who need medical assistance to achieve pregnancy and those who need intervention to stimulate milk flow for breastfeeding.

Unfortunately, medical professionals, such as Pat, who want to support new moms in their breastfeeding must also contend with the looming presence of corporate giants who stand to make a lot of money if mom chooses formula. Georgetown University pediatrics professor Naomi Baumslag writes that for each dollar charged for formula, only 16 cents is spent on production and delivery.[19] Cans of formula generally sell for around $20.00 each. So a company will spend $3.20 making the product and getting it to the store shelf. The remaining $16.80 per can buys these formula companies a lot of advertising and marketing muscle and adds to their cushy profit. Through years of relentless advertising, insinuating themselves into medical groups, and giving new parents free product and coupons, they have managed to convince a lot of us that formula-feeding is the way to go.

Think about the coupons, free cans of formula, diaper bags, and other paraphernalia that many new mothers are given upon discharge from the maternity ward. "Hospitals don't normally give things away," writes Ruth A. Lawrence, professor of pediatrics at the University of Rochester School of Medicine and the chair of the American Academy of Pediatrics (AAP) section on breastfeeding. "When they send you home, they don't give you medicines

and bandages. This is obviously promoted by the formula companies. Free stuff implies an endorsement."

Some places are cracking down on this. Hospitals in California, Colorado, Texas, and Massachusetts have enacted bans on
the blatant distribution of formula samples to new mothers. In
2007, Mayor Michael Bloomberg enacted a similar prohibition
regarding the 11 hospitals in the New York City Public Hospital
system, where 21,000 babies are born each year. In a concentrated effort to increase the rate of breastfeeding in that city,
new moms now receive diaper bags that contain breast milk
bottle coolers and a T-shirt for the baby that reads "I Eat at
Mom's."

"Foul," cried some critics, making the ridiculous point that
this move is "unfair to low-income mothers." (And just what,
one might ask, is fair about offering promotional materials for
high-priced products to low-income people, when there is a better alternative available for free?) Always on the lookout for
ways to endear themselves to the medical community, formula
companies give $1 million each year to the American Academy
of Pediatrics, give thousands of dollars in research grants and
aid to physicians, dietitians, and other health professionals, and
provided $3 million in assistance for the construction of a new
AAP headquarters building.[20] All of this so that your doctor, or
your new child's doctor, will "support you in your decision" to
formula-feed.

I'll get off my soapbox now and get on to my second point.
Beyond what I've already said, I'm going to stay out of the whole
medical side of the breast milk–formula debate because I am simply not qualified to go there. My concern, after all, is how what
we put in our children's mouths affects the development of their
sense of taste and, later, food choice and acceptance. And there is
more than enough to work with on the subject of breastfeeding
and taste, without engaging in the medical side of the issue.

Much of the research pertaining to the influence of expectant moms' diets on their infant's food choices applies directly to breastfeeding as well. Any new mother who has seen her infant cry hysterically and recoil from stomach gas pains, only to be told by the pediatrician to cut out dairy products and certain other foods, like broccoli, from her own diet while breastfeeding, knows the impact that a mother's diet has on a breastfeeding baby. Is it such a stretch to believe that a well-balanced and flavorful diet also has the same power to influence a baby's food preferences positively?

"One of the greatest benefits that breast milk has over formula is that its nutrient content varies throughout the day, to give the infant exactly what he needs," says Pat Shelly. "Levels of fat and protein, for example, tend to be higher later in the day and rise with frequency of nursing." Might the flavor of the breast milk— the way that it tastes and is received by the baby—also fluctuate in this way? "Oh yes," she affirms. "In fact, we've had toddlers who are being breastfed comment on changes in the taste of the milk, based on what their mother has been eating."

Again, scientific evidence backs this up. Jean Skinner and Betty Ruth Carruth, referring to another study conducted at Monell, write that "both fruit variety and exposures in infancy are significant predictors of fruit variety scores in the school-aged child, again emphasizing the importance of early experiences with later eating patterns. This finding is consistent with the notion that infants' experiences with breast milk enhance their exposure [to] and thus their acceptance of a wide variety of flavors."[21]

Julie Mennella saw similar results in a study that evaluated the effects of breastfeeding on acceptance of fruit and green vegetables by older infants. Forty-five four-to-eight-month-old infants, nineteen of whom were breastfed, were given either green beans or green beans and peaches to eat. The babies who were breastfed liked the peaches better, as did their mothers, who ate more fruits in general than did mothers who formula-fed. And although the formula-feeding moms ate more green beans, their babies did not accept this vegetable more readily.[22]

And for further evidence, consider this: why is it that when they are ready to learn to eat, Asian babies readily accept Asian foods, babies from the Middle East their own native cuisines, and many American babies . . . well, a lot of them just don't get aggressively-spiced foods very early. Cultural differences in eating definitely come into play here. Long before she can teach her children to cook, a mother gives her kids a lesson in native food cuisines and traditions. Mom's diet while breastfeeding is the first way that babies experience these flavors.

With this in mind, treat yourself to a wide abundance of your favorite flavors and more while pregnant and breastfeeding. Mexican, Thai, Indian, Mediterranean, African; enjoy whatever you like, and know that Baby will, too. If you're cooking for yourself, add a wide variety of herbs and spices to your meal. Dill, anise, sage, oregano, mint, garlic, and many others all provide distinct flavor profiles that you can incorporate second-hand into Baby's milk. While salty and sweet may come naturally, don't forget to add sharp or bitter-flavored foods to your menu, things like broccoli, arugula, and spinach. At the very least, you can have some fun with this and enjoy some good eating yourself. And at most, you are exposing your newborn to an abundance of flavors and setting the stage for the development of a broad palate.

One caveat to remember to increase the odds of success: you need to be eating these foods not only early, but also often. "Breastfeeding confers an advantage in initial acceptance of a food, but only if mothers eat the food regularly," write Mennella and colleague Catherine Forestell.[23]

Formula, obviously, does not provide Baby with any comparable variation in flavor. How would you like it if you had to eat the same single piece of food, day after day, night after night, for five or six months? "In the lactation field, we call formula 'artificial infant milk,'" says Pat Shelly. "Formula is usually made from broken-down cow's milk, along with added vitamins, minerals, and algae. Other formulas sometimes used for more sensitive babies are made from soy and hydrolyzed (broken-down) proteins." The flavor profile of most infant formulas is similar to breast milk: sweet.

If you are going the formula route for whatever reason, are there steps that you can take to broaden the flavor experience? Yes, say researchers at Monell, who found that the type of formula fed to babies influences the child's flavor preferences for foods, both immediately and several years down the road. Their work shows that the less sweet the formula you give Baby, the better luck you may have getting her to like foods that are not sweet in the years to come.

Take two groups of babies, both age six to eleven months, one on a diet of sweet-flavored, milk-based formula, the second drinking a protein formula that has more of a sulfur taste, similar to broccoli. Researchers observed their initial reactions to carrots and to a combination of broccoli and cauliflower. You would think that the milk formula babies would like the sweeter carrots, and the protein formula babies would like the broccoli/cauliflower, right? But the opposite was true. Both groups liked the carrots, but the protein formula–fed babies ate much less of the broccoli and cauliflower mixture.

The Monell group calls this a "sensory specific satiety following repeated exposure to a particular flavor in milk."[24] In other words, when the babies got used to that bitter flavor in their milk, initially they only wanted it in that form. It would take some time before they were eager to accept it as food.

However, what happens when these babies grow up to be toddlers or preschoolers? Can you still see the effects of their formula consumption? Well, it appears that formula type influenced children's flavor preferences when tested several years later. Children who had consumed the more bitter-tasting protein-based formulas were more predisposed to like sour juices and broccoli than were the milk-based-formula-fed kids.[25] So the children ended up preferring foods with flavor reminiscent of the formula that they drank as babies.

Spin the Bottle

"I've only given my baby son a bottle maybe five times in his whole life. I'm a stay-at-home mom so I've been lazy about pumping. However, I have some big events coming up like a wedding and some dental surgery, so I really need for him to learn to supplement with a bottle. At the rate I'm going, I'm afraid I'll never get out of the house alone!"
Carly, mom to a seven-month-old

Even if you're breastfeeding exclusively, and obviously if you're not, you'll probably want to teach Baby to drink milk from bottles. You might manage to be with your baby around the clock for the first weeks or few months, but, eventually, there will come a time when you'll want or need to be away, and she will need to be fed breast milk or formula from a bottle.

I have heard of many babies who are so used to being breastfed that they have a hard time learning to accept bottles. I'm sure the switch is a bit of a shock to them; after all, they are used to a warm, soft nipple in which they can control the speed of flow of the milk, and then they are asked to try something harder, colder, and made of plastic. So it may take more than one attempt at bottle feeding before Baby gets the hang of it and can be convinced that this is what he is going to have to do. Just keep at it; bottle-feeding is another skill that Baby will eventually master. Let him practice at one or two feedings a day until he really gets good at it.

And not long after Baby masters this one, it may be time to move on to sippy cups. Most pediatricians will tell you that Baby should be off of the bottle by her first birthday, or shortly thereafter. Teaching Baby the skills that she will need for proper drinking and eating is an important developmental milestone, so don't drag your feet too long on this one. An earlier transition is actually easier than a delayed one, as bottle habits only get more ingrained over time. You may also notice that Baby is drinking a little less milk at this point; that's normal, because more of her calories and nutrients are now coming from food.

Finally, keep this last tip in mind: *never* let Baby take a bottle to bed. It's so tempting, I know, when he needs a little help in getting to sleep, but a bottle in bed is a bad habit to get into and even a couple of exceptions can lead to future expectations. Pediatricians will tell you not to do this because it is bad for Baby's developing teeth. I'm going to give you another reason: this is a first step in helping Baby to understand that meals and snacks happen according to a set schedule, in a regular time and place, and are not nibbled along as a source of comfort or as a sleep aid. Do you want your preschooler to be snacking all over the house, or your teenager to leave dirty dishes in his room? In the interest of consistency, give him the message now, a few years in advance. We respect food. We enjoy food, in its proper place.

Breastfeeding: A Final Encouragement

"I work at a medical testing and research lab that doesn't provide a mother's nursing room. So when I went back to work and started pumping, I looked for the most private area that I could find. I finally

*settled on a refrigerated specimen storage room. Several times a day,
I would sit in a dark room among the tissue samples and vials of body
fluids to pump. It was actually quite peaceful."*
New mom's posting on parenting Web site, when asked
about "the most unusual place you've pumped"

One of the great benefits of being a new mother is that you realize that, very quickly, you're going to make a lot of new friends.

After the birth of first son Willie, I so looked forward to the meetings of the new moms' groups that I joined, as places to swap advice and stories and receive loads of sympathetic encouragement when things were getting difficult. Women who just one month earlier had been leading meetings in corporate boardrooms and arguing cases in courtrooms now gathered eagerly in dingy church basements, discussing nighttime feeding schedules and numbers of dirty diapers produced each day. No one cared that we hadn't washed our hair in a week. Nothing promotes female bonding like this kind of situation.

And at these gathering the stories about the trials and tribulations of breastfeeding would flow, sometimes with tears, but more often with laughter as we outdid each other with tales of "you're not going to believe what happened to me." Some women (and babies) had real struggles learning to breastfeed, for others it was easier. But we all needed encouragement at various points to continue, as we came to recognize what a commitment of time and energy breastfeeding is. I still remember one of the moms stating very clearly that she had "almost quit" several times, but stuck it out with the realization that there would be many, many more times in the long road of parenthood that lay ahead that she would have to choose between doing what was expedient at the moment and doing what was in the long-term best interest of her child.

"Today it's throwing in the towel and turning to formula; in a couple of years it will be giving in and feeding her hot dogs every night because that's what she wants to eat," this new mom said. "There's always an easier way for me, but that doesn't mean it's the best for my kid."

This mother raises a very wise point, one that I wish the research community would take some interest in. I could find no credible papers drawing a direct link between consuming formula as an infant and turning out to be a Picky Eater as a toddler or preschooler. In other words, if that is what happens, medical science would probably say it's purely a coincidence. However, I'm going to go out on a limb here and say that, from observational evidence alone, I do think there is some correlation between being formula-fed rather than breastfed as a baby and growing into a young child who will eat only a narrow range of foods. And that cause is not a scientific one, necessarily, but a reflection of parental attitudes and actions on feeding.

If you're a parent who, for whatever reason, makes the choice for formula-feeding over breastfeeding, then you are saying that you are convinced that formula products are, at minimum, safe to consume and nutritionally sound. You have implicitly accepted the position statements of the medical community (American Academy of Pediatrics), the federal government (Food and Drug Administration), and the corporate marketing departments behind the products. Logic may tell you that "natural is better," but chances are, you won't even stop to think about it.

And thus you have unknowingly taken the first step in succumbing to the prevailing attitude of many American parents about the way that their kids eat. That attitude is: "If 'They' sell it or market it for babies/toddlers/children/young adults, then it's not only good for kids—it is what they are supposed to have." Starting now, at the formula stage, this is the parental mindset that you will most often encounter, as your child's eating progresses to baby foods, toddler products, kiddie snacks, children's menus, fast foods, sodas and energy drinks, and probably beyond. Parents who want to avoid these generic-tasting products in favor of better quality and better-flavored foods for their kids will have some tough times. But doing so may allow you to reap the benefit of having a child who is more adaptable when it comes to foods, more willing to try new things, and more apt to enjoy meals in a healthful way.

So, if you're convinced that breastfeeding is the way to go and you want to plug along with it, I will tell you that some of the best encouragement I can give you is to learn to take the whole process with a bit of humor. I mean, you cannot make up the crazy things that happened to some of the women I talked to, when I asked for their best breastfeeding stories.

One woman told me about pumping in an airplane bathroom, using a hand-held, battery operated pump. A man (of course) waiting outside of the bathroom door heard the strange whirring sound of the pump and alerted a flight attendant that something suspicious was going on in the bathroom. "He probably thought I was making a bomb. So I had no choice but to yell 'I'm breastfeeding and I'm pumping' when the flight attendant knocked on the door to ask what I was doing in the bathroom," this mom said. "The entire back half of the plane witnessed this encounter."

Another friend told of investing in an expensive carrying case for her breast pump, one that looked just like a designer briefcase. She thought it would be perfect for toting the thing back and forth once she returned to work. Apparently, it was too attractive: her husband inadvertently picked it up on his way out to a client presentation, mistaking it for his own bag that contained a million-dollar contract proposal. Whoops!

Other women told me about sneaking out to rest rooms to pump during business meetings, pumping in a car while in the parking lot of a fancy California winery before a wine-tasting tour, and during intermissions of theatrical performances. One friend said that her biggest disaster came when she was on a four-day business trip. She had religiously pumped several times each day, storing every precious drop to take home to her baby. She said that she was about halfway to the airport for the return trip when she realized that in her haste to check out, she had left six bottles of milk in the mini-bar refrigerator of her Ritz-Carlton hotel room. (Sorry about that, next guest!)

So you see, a bit of stress, a little anxiety, and a few good laughs do come with the territory. Welcome to parenthood!

What I've Learned

— Generally, kids who have broad and varied diets and adventuresome attitudes toward food live with parents who feel and behave that way. If you're a picky or limited eater yourself, chances are very good that your kids will be as well. Only it will seem worse with them, because as an adult, you've learned to adapt your finickiness to fit in with the rest of the world and know better than to ask for a hot dog at a business banquet!

— Paying attention to diet during pregnancy and lactation can really pay off, and not just in nutritional and health benefits. Clear scientific evidence shows that mom's diet will eventually affect baby's eating and taste preferences.

— Breastfeeding can be tough, but it is so, so worthwhile, in so many ways. Trust me on this one: you will be glad that you stuck it out. And although you may get reassurances to the contrary from people or organizations that have some vested interest in the formula industry, formula-feeding is definitely a second-place alternative.

— Sometimes humor really is the best medicine. Laugh a little, with Baby and at yourself. You can do this.

CHAPTER 4

⌘

"Into the Mouths of Babes": First Foods

S omewhere around the fourth month of your child's life—perhaps a bit later, especially if Baby was premature— it will be time to start on what we all lovingly refer to as "solid foods," the first "baby" step on the road to real eating. And as you will discover in just about all areas of parenting, there is no lack of opinion on when and how this should be done. (And you thought you got a lot of free advice during pregnancy. Just wait!)

Many new parents fret endlessly about the "right" time to start these feedings, as though there were one correct, predetermined hour or day that they must not miss in their child's development process. Complicating this decision is the abundance of mixed messages that you will find on the topic if you start researching: some parenting books say one thing, Web sites may say another, and your pediatrician may just give a vague "you'll know when the time comes" type of response to your queries. (Your own parents or in-laws may wonder what you're waiting for; a couple of generations ago, babies started on solids earlier than they typically do now. And in many parts of the world, early introduction to solids is still the norm.)

You can be sure that the baby food manufacturing companies, if you're interested in their opinion, want your child eating solids as soon as possible, and why not? In their worldview, a new little consumer has been born. These are the "helpful" people who produce much of the written literature that is distributed by your pediatrician, as well as "informational" Web sites and toll-free telephone numbers for free consultations on feeding questions. So keep in mind their mercenary perspective, and be just a bit skeptical of baby food packaging information that says that cereals are for infants who have doubled their birth weight and weigh at least 13 pounds. In William's case, that would have been at just under four months, and in Daniel's, barely three. Neither of my kids was ready to start solids at those prescribed times. (To be fair, these manufacturers do note that a baby also (1) should be able to sit supported, and (2) still be hungry after ten breastfeeding sessions or consuming 32 ounces of formula a day, before he or she is ready for the cereals.)

Just remember that breast milk and/or formula provide all of the necessary nutritional elements needed for the first six to nine months of life. The solid foods that you start adding to the diet before that time provide some supplemental vitamins and minerals, of course, but solids become the primary source of nutrients only gradually. In these first few weeks of soft solids, a major goal is simply to teach Baby the how-tos of taking something new into the mouth, tasting, and then swallowing it.

With that in mind, you should realize that determining when to move on to "the hard stuff" becomes more of an art than a science. If you start too early and Baby is incapable of performing the physical requirements of processing food in the mouth and then swallowing, you run the risk of choking and presenting substances that may be too advanced for a baby's digestive system. But wait too late, and it becomes more difficult to teach these new skills, and your child will start missing out on important nutrients. Equally important, there is some evidence that a late start on solid foods—after about seven months of age—can result in a narrower range of accepted foods throughout childhood. "There needs to be more research done on this," says Elizabeth Cashdan, PhD, an anthropologist at the University of Utah who has studied food acceptance and aversions in young children. "But from the few studies that have been done on Western diets and culture, we know that introducing solids at a late age can be expected to cause a reduction in diet breadth."[26]

To that, Dr. Sydney Spiesel, a Connecticut pediatrician, professor at Yale Medical School, and medical columnist at Slate.com, adds, "I worry most about children who start solid foods on the later end; those who are still eating soft purées late into infancy. They are missing some important development skills in learning how to eat."

The one caution I offer is not to make your decision on this based solely on the "what's easiest for me" criteria. Many moms are fully into the swing of nursing at this point and may find it less of a hassle to just keep breastfeeding exclusively, rather than moving on to the solids stage. Others are so desperate for a full night's sleep that they want to start solids on the early side, relying on the old wives' tale—an incorrect one, by the way—that a tummy full of solid food will keep Baby sleeping longer. Using personal convenience as the major determinant can lead you down the wrong path.

The best bet is not to sweat over it, ask your pediatrician for input, and let your baby lead the way. By his actions, he will "tell" you when the time is right.

Look at this as another one of those wonderfully awe-inspiring times that you will experience with your child during his first year of life. Start allowing Baby to come to the dinner table with you—sitting in your lap, or in a highchair or bouncy chair placed nearby—and watch his reaction. All of a sudden, it will seem, he will be *interested* in your eating. He will hear the laughter and conversation of the group, and want to take part. He may stare intensely at the food on your plate, following every step as you cut it up, put it on a fork and eat. He may start reaching out to grab a napkin or spoon, or even plop a chubby hand in the middle of your pile of green beans. In babyspeak, he's saying, "Hey, that looks like fun! I want to try it!"

Open Wide!

"I used to try to wipe the cereal off of his face as he was eating his meal, but now I've realized that's futile, because with every bite, some ends up in his hair or on his chin or neck. He's a mess by the time he finishes eating, but he looks happy so I know that some of it must be getting into his stomach!"
Jill, mother of a five-month-old

Usually, the first solid food of choice is infant cereal, recommended by most pediatricians as the preferred starter food because it is easy for babies to digest and poses little risk of allergic reaction. (There are several brands and many flavor varieties on the market, including some made with organic flours. They all provide roughly identical nutritional profiles in terms of calories and ingredients, though some are higher in sugar content than others.) Stick to the plain flavors, such as rice, wheat, barley, and mixed grains cereals, as opposed to the ones with banana flakes, apple flakes, or any sort of added fruit flavor. Those with "fruit" additions usually also have a slightly higher sugar content, and it adds nothing to the product but preserved fruit flavor. When the time comes to add some flavor to Baby's rice cereal, it's much better to wait until she can handle real fruits.

You'll quickly develop your own routine of how to best go about feeding your baby.

You probably received some of those cute little dishes and tiny baby feeding spoons at a baby shower or when your child was born; pull these out, or just use any small bowl or demi-tasse spoon. Regular teaspoons are too big for the child's mouth at this point and should only be used in a pinch, such as when you're away from home and have forgotten to stash the baby spoon in a diaper bag. Pour one to two tablespoons of the cereal into the bowl and stir in three or four tablespoons of water, breast milk, or formula. The consistency of the mixture should be very moist and almost liquid, but not runny.

Put a little bit of infant cereal on the tip of the spoon and offer it to your child. The first reaction may well resemble a "what in the heck is this?" response. After all, your baby has been eating one food—milk—for all of his or her short life. (And if he has been formula-fed, it's been a very consistent product with virtually no variation in taste for all these months.) Don't be surprised if some of the cereal comes back out, or if baby appears to be actually spitting it out. This is a reflex of the tongue that will disappear as she grows and understands the process. It does not mean that Baby doesn't like the food! (Note: if this tongue thrusting-out reflex is strong and continues over several tries, stop and wait a week or two before trying again. It could mean that your baby is simply not ready to attempt regular eating.)

Some parents ask about the need to heat the cereal; I think this is another bad piece of information from the manufacturing companies. Their packaging gives directions on how to microwave the food, and suggests that the cereal be mixed with warmed liquid. If Baby is accustomed to warm food (as in body temperature breast milk or warmed formula), this is a good time to let her know that food doesn't always have to be presented in one way to taste good. You're setting yourself up for problems down the road if Baby comes to expect food always served at a consistent temperature.

For at least the first few eating sessions, use breast milk, water, or formula to liquefy the cereals, as your baby is already familiar with the taste of these. Later, you can try chicken stock or vegetable broth for added flavor. Some packages list "infant juice" as an acceptable mixer—another big mistake if you are at all concerned about the amount of sweet foods that your child consumes, or will be consuming as he grows. Again, why would you want to teach a child now that food is supposed to be sweet? (Answer from the manufacturer: because we want to sell you more baby juice! And eventually, sweetened kid's cereals, candy, soft drinks . . . see where this is going?)

The fact that there is, for the first time, a little choice in foods is enough for now, so take advantage of it. Buy a box of each type of cereal (rice, oatmeal, barley, mixed grains), introduce them to the diet one at a time according to your pediatrician's directions, and then start combining and mixing it up a bit to give the baby a sense of flavor variation.

The first feedings with a new baby are special times that many new parents love to document with a camera. These are wonderful moments, and it's fun to approach them as such: baby is taking a first tentative step towards something that you hope he or she will approach with relish for a lifetime. Parents or caregivers can start now to create an association between "food" and "pleasure." Make it a point to smile at your baby while feeding her. Talk to her about what she's doing. And love the smiles that you will get in return.

Moving On to the Tasty Stuff

"My daughter will eat puréed foods if she's the only one eating, but if we're all having dinner or another meal together, she will shout and scream until she's given bites of what we're having. Even without teeth, she does a great job of gumming down rice, berries, chicken, asparagus—basically, whatever we're having."
Suzette, mother of an eight-month-old

"I remember with both of my kids, when they were six or seven months old, I was cooking braised meats, like braised osso bucco or short ribs. Very soft meats, cut up small. That was probably both of my children's first baby food."
Chef Robbie Lewis, Bacar Restaurant, San Francisco

So it's a few weeks down the road, and Baby seems to have mastered the range of cereals. Now you can get ready to progress to adult foods—mashed, puréed, and otherwise mangled into such a form that adults would not recognize them, of course. When to step up to more flavorful offerings? Dr. Sydney Spiesel has an interesting observation, albeit, he says, an anecdotal one, formed from observing many babies in his practice over the years.

"Until the age of about five and a half months, most babies prefer to eat what we adults would call very bland flavors, like those found in formula, breast milk, and infant cereals," Spiesel says. "I suspect that this is nature's way of protecting them from ingesting a harmful substance, most of which are bitter tasting or at least a lot stronger in taste.

"But at almost precisely the age of five and a half months (about 24–25 weeks), babies suddenly seem to acquire an interest in more strongly flavored and even spicy foods. And by the six-month mark, babies seem to actively search out these better-tasting foods."

Coincidentally, I spoke with Dr. Spiesel on the telephone during the week that my Daniel turned six months old. And that was exactly the week that Daniel's interest in solid foods seemed to come alive. Sitting in my lap at the dinner table, he flailed his hands, stretched across the table to touch a salad bowl and sent the unmistakable message that he was hungry for the good stuff. Daniel had always been a healthy eater, but that was the point that we knew that he was ready for something more than rice cereal. "I'm not surprised," Dr. Spiesel told me. "I see that all the time."

Many people and books will tell you to introduce vegetables, such as sweet potatoes, peas, green beans, and squash, first, and then proceed to the sweeter fruits, such as bananas, pears, and apples. The assumption is that since "sweet" will be the preferred flavor, it will be harder to get a baby to accept stronger-tasting vegetables if he has become accustomed to fruits. While this may be a good idea, and there is certainly nothing wrong with introducing vegetables first, I find the general theory to be an admission of how much we've all bought into the idea that every child will automatically insist on "sweet" every time, and must somehow be protected from himself and coerced into eating those horrible vegetables. This practice doesn't make a lot of sense, if you stop to think about it: even if you do give vegetables first and then move onto fruits, if this guideline is so correct, then why wouldn't Baby refuse to eat a vegetable ever again, once he's tasted that fantastic fruit?

Whether or not you realize it, your child has already had quite the mouthful of sweetness at this point, as both breast milk and formula have a sweet flavor. It is quite possible, then, that babies appear to accept fruits more readily at this point because the sweet flavor is more familiar. An introduction of stronger or bitter-tasting vegetables may elicit a startled look from Baby because he simply hasn't experienced this flavor in the past, especially to this intensity.

Start out slowly, following your doctor's directions to introduce just one food at a time and spread out over several days, to stay on the watch for potential food allergies. Put the foods in a food processor or blender, give them a good whirl, and they are ready to go, eaten as is or mixed in with a cereal that is already familiar. Most important: enjoy this stage and, if you're a food-lover yourself, revel in it! Your child is going to experience, for the first time, what an apple or a sweet potato tastes like, and learn that foods have different colors, aromas, and flavors. What a wonderful process to be witness to! My husband, who grew up in the Pennsylvania apple country and still eats an apple a day if he has one available, couldn't wait to see our kids' reactions to their first bite of this fruit that we hope will be a big part of their diets for the rest of their lives.

Sometimes when trying something new, Baby will turn up her nose at the food, making a little pucker face that seems to be saying "Yuck!" She may spit some or all of it out of her mouth, giving the distinct impression that this food choice is not a winner. You will probably see this many times as you introduce new foods, but here is an important point in mind: *this reaction does not mean that she does not like the food being offered!*

Leann L. Birch, PhD, is a psychologist at Pennsylvania State University who has devoted much of her academic career to research on the development of children's food-acceptance patterns. In a 1995 study on this topic, she notes that the taste system is functional at birth and that newborns show reflexive facial expressions elicited by basic tastes. The interesting thing, however, is adults' and caregivers' responses to these expressions. "She likes it!" we tend to exclaim when an infant tries something sweet and responds with a smile; or, "Oh, he doesn't like that" is the natural first reaction to a puckered face that may follow a first taste of a bitter or sour flavor. The problem is, Birch notes, we don't realize that these facial expressions are simply reflexes, "built-in" from birth.[27]

"Caregivers interpret the infant's facial and gestural responses to foods and make decisions about whether to continue feeding a food, to stop the feeding, or to try a different food," Birch writes in this fascinating study called *Children's Eating: The Development of Food-Acceptance Patterns*. "The fact that these early responses to the basic tastes are reflexive ones suggests that food acceptance patterns may be 'hardwired'—fixed and difficult to change, but research on the development of children's food-acceptance patterns reveals that this is not the case." The positive responses to sweetness and the visual rejection of bitter and sour are 'built-in,' writes Dr. Birch, but from very early in life, even responses to these basic tastes will change with Baby's repeated experience with food and eating.

As variety develops in Baby's diet, you can begin to phase out the infant cereals. When you recognize that you are just using cereals as a thickening agent for other foods, it is a good time to drop them permanently from the menu. Meats, such as chicken, pork, and beef, are usually added to the diet a little later, around seven or eight months. From there, it's on to foods with a bit of texture; finger foods such as crackers, pieces of bread, cut-up chicken, or chunks of cheese. You will soon find that Baby wants to join you in just about everything that you are eating.

Also, as your infant gets older, he will probably want to be more involved in the feeding process, grabbing spoons from you to try to self-feed, for example, or insisting on touching and examining every bit of food before putting it into her mouth. You may find this to be either funny or maddening, depending on the mood you're in, the level of messiness, and the time that it takes to complete a feeding. Try to remain sane throughout this period, and remember that this is the way that Baby can best explore her cuisine options. Different foods have different colors and textures—how interesting! Cheerios or raisins scatter when dropped to the floor, while grape slices and watermelon pieces splatter! Meat can be pulled apart, mashed potatoes smear, peas smash!

Don't be afraid to go your own way, plot a course that works for you and your baby, and have a little fun with it. Other than shellfish, nuts, and citrus fruits (foods that the American Academy of Pediatrics recommends avoiding for the first year of life), the sky—or your pantry, refrigerator, or restaurant menu—is the limit on what Baby can and should eat. And remember: babies under the age of one are more likely to accept new foods on the first or second try. If you want him to love sweet potatoes (or sautéed collard greens or your favorite Thai food dish), don't wait until he hits the predictably cantankerous toddler stage to give those more intensely flavored foods a try. Introducing a range of new foods "works best if initiated when the child first begins to try new foods, during late infancy prior to the increased autonomy and independence of the toddler period," writes Birch.[28]

Repeat, Repeat, Repeat

"(When my kids were small), my thing was always having a lot of variety, re-introducing things, and having a good balance between fruits and vegetables."
Chef Barbara Black, Black Salt Restaurant, Washington, D.C.,
mother of two young boys

So it's not going so swimmingly at your house? Don't think you're alone; various studies that I consulted said that as many as 25% of infants have some sort of feeding problem, ranging from eating too little, to accepting only a limited number of foods, to objectionable mealtime behaviors, to just downright bizarre eating habits. The good news is that in the vast majority of cases these issues can be resolved, or at least managed, over time, with a little persistence from mom and dad.

Dr. Birch's research asks the question: which of the many dimensions of foods are most important in forming children's food preferences? Food flavor, texture, color, and temperature are all possible responses. But it turns out that one of the most important factors in whether or not a child liked a particular food item was whether or not he had eaten it before. "Children tend to prefer foods that are familiar over those that are not," writes Dr. Birch. "This is independent of the foods' sensory characteristics."[29]

All foods are new to children at some point. Like all other mammals, we begin life with a milk diet and gradually progress to more hearty fare. And the way that we do that, more often than not, is to taste and taste and taste again a particular food, until it becomes a regular and accepted part of our diet. As exposure to a new food increases, so does the child's acceptance of that food.

This is one of those things that you just have to stick with, even if and when the going gets rough. Merely having the child look at or smell the new food is not enough, Birch writes; children must actually repeatedly sample the food. And by "repeatedly" she does not mean a couple of tastings, followed by adamant refusals, followed by a parental "never again." No, "repeatedly" in this instance translates to up to fifteen separate eating occasions. Skinner and Carruth concur: "Studies have shown that frequency of exposure is a factor in food acceptance, suggesting that parents and caregivers should not rely on one or two rejections to determine if the child will or will not like and eat a food."[30]

Birch recommends a schedule that includes two opportunities to try a given new food each week. There should be an expectation from you, the parent, that Baby will try all new foods when offered. She also points out that this policy works best at this stage, during late infancy. Wait too long and you'll have a more independent Toddler on your hands. And that may call for a whole new strategy to continue guiding the development of a broad palate.

I've recently had the good fortune of being able to try out this advice first-hand, as baby Daniel has developed into a self-feeder.

From the start, it was apparent that although he was an excellent early eater (in terms of volume of food consumed), he was going to be a bit more finicky about new foods than William had been. "What to do?" I wondered more than once; I can't have a potential Picky Eater on my hands! So I waited him out, and in some cases, I'm still waiting him out, introducing again and again the foods that he has been reluctant to accept. Slowly, it's working. As an example, he's gone from completely rejecting the canned tuna in tuna salads (but loving grilled tuna filets), to allowing spoonfuls to stay on his high chair tray, to actually picking them up and giving them a try. Sometimes, the bites come back out. But then we try again, and eventually, he gets it.

All I can recommend at this point is just keep at it. Serve rejected foods again and then again, after a few days or a week or so. One of the biggest feeding mistakes that parents make at this point, I think, is to swear off a food (or many foods) "forever," just because Baby doesn't appear to like them once or twice. Remember the research: as many as fifteen failed attempts before success is not uncommon for some children and some foods. Just keep trying, and take advantage of this time when she can't yet verbally refuse!

As Baby's teeth grow in, add to the texture complexity in food choices. Babies and toddlers have to be taught how to take small bites and chew their food; their tendency is to stuff large portions into their mouths. Show them at an early stage how to chew food properly. Small teaspoons or standard baby-food spoons are particularly helpful in this endeavor. Get right down in his face, at eye-level, and show him a "chewing" motion. You'll be surprised at how quickly Baby will pick it up.

There is a big difference between Baby not taking immediately to a new food—putting it in and out of his mouth with a little uncertainly, perhaps because he is not really hungry at the moment—and stopping his feeding altogether because he has had enough to eat. This is another one of those things in which parents seem to intuitively learn how to read Baby's cues. If he has been eating heartily and all of a sudden turns away, seems distracted, or, in the case of a more dramatic baby, actually starts shoving the spoon back at you, take it to mean that he has had enough for this feeding session. Even if it seems to you like he didn't eat very much, just stop, respect what he is trying to tell you, and pick it up again later, when he makes it clear that he is hungry.

Weight management expert Pat Harper, RD, of the University of Pittsburgh, is the former chief dietitian at the Children's Hospital in Buffalo, New York. Now working with adults in weight-loss programs, Pat has seen the full spectrum of our nation's obesity problems, and thinks that some weight management problems encountered later in life could have roots in childhood feeding patterns. "Think of what it would be like if you couldn't speak and relied on someone else to feed you," Pat said. "When you had enough to eat, you couldn't say so in words, but tried to signal that you were full by turning your head or pushing the food away. But no matter how you objected, the person kept feeding you, almost forcing you to eat and ignoring your wishes. Then imagine that you suddenly learned how to communicate in words. After months and months of frustration, your first instinct would be to shout 'NO' when confronted with food when you'd had enough or didn't want to eat something."

"That's how it is with toddlers," she continued. "They find a voice by speaking or acting out during meals, now that they are able to express the frustrations with food that they have been experiencing all along, since babyhood. The food jags and rebellion that are common in the 'terrible twos' may just be a reaction to the feeling of being 'force-fed' before they could talk."

A final feeding tip: don't forget the importance of personal interaction with your baby during feeding time. "Yum, Yum, Yum!" you can remind him, while smiling and even taking bites of the food yourself. This is his first introduction to conversation at the dinner table, and he is most likely to respond with glee and try new foods willingly if he sees that you are interested in the food yourself. More research has found that children's willingness to taste offered foods is positively influenced by the adults tasting the food before offering it to them.[31]

Baby Daniel's first word was all about food. He started saying "good" (actually, more like "gu"), with a big smile on his face and an occasional clapping of his hands. I, as his mother, immediately knew that this was his complement to the chef! Lately, he's added a little grunt and an opening and closing of his fists to the repertoire; I have come to recognize these gestures as meaning "keep the food coming."

If you view this stage of life as an opportunity to begin to develop your child's palate, so that he or she can start learning that eating is about enjoyment and health, then realize that much more important than the precise order of introduction of individual foods is the *flavor* of each item that Baby is being exposed to. And that's where this gets really interesting.

Baby Foods: Yours or Theirs

"[When my boys were babies], I used to give them scraped apples and avocadoes. We always made their baby food, and added a little butter and even some salt to season it. It's fresher and healthier than what's in a jar."
Chef Marc Collins, Circa 1886 Restaurant, Charleston, SC, father of two young boys

Compared to all the years ahead in which you will be preparing meals for your child, it is now that cooking for him will be the easiest, the least expensive, and probably the most gratifying. Yes, there is a wide range of suitable baby foods available commercially, and these are good to have on hand in a pinch. But before you spend too much time and money stocking up in the baby food aisle of the grocery store, give some thought to the merits of making your child's first foods the homemade variety.

The purpose of this book—a purpose that distinguishes it from the many other books available on feeding young children—is to present to parents and caregivers the idea that just about any child can be taught to prefer healthful, fresh "real" foods, over more standard American "kid fare." For that reason, I'll start with a focus on the taste of baby foods, commercial versus homemade, as a primary reason to forgo the former in favor of the latter. There are other reasons to do that, too, that are presented here, but my main focus is flavor. To get Baby's little palate off to the right start, nothing beats the flavor exposure he will get from real home cooking.

When I was interviewing chefs for this book, asking them to tell us all what they feed or fed their own babies, one of them asked me point-blank about commercial baby food: "Have you ever tasted that stuff?" I had to admit that I had not. My Willie had certainly had his share of store-bought baby food during his infancy, interspersed, as I recalled, with homemade purées and concoctions as often as I took the time to prepare them. With Baby Daniel coming along, this seemed like the perfect opportunity to try for myself the baby food products that I and countless thousands of other mothers routinely give their infants. I mean, if he is going to eat it on a daily basis, shouldn't I be willing to at least give it a little try?

So under the proposition of "taking one for the team," I conducted a taste test of many of the commercial baby foods that you will find at the grocery store. (I did this so that you don't have to!) A group of food-loving friends—all parents, and one a chef—and I sampled a wide range of foods from all of the leading brands, organic and non-organic, from the starter foods (generally labeled as "Ones"), through the product lines offered for older infants (labeled something like "Twos" or "Threes"). I also prepared fresh, homemade varieties of the same foods, to have a reference point for what the foods "should" taste like.

What we found is not likely to be a big surprise to anyone. In a nutshell, there is simply no quality equivalency in the taste and flavor of the commercial products, presented alongside the same foods prepared at home. The color comparison was the first giveaway in predicting the results of this little experiment. Next to the vibrant hues of the homemade mashes, the commercial sweet potatoes, peas, green beans, bananas, and others were dull and dark-looking. And except for the pungent bananas, there was no discernible aroma to any of the store-bought products, certainly not any that was an identifying feature.

In fact, the greatest revelation was exactly how far the store-bought products are from replicating the taste of fresh food. Sampled together, the homemade and the purchased are not even close.

To give you an idea of what Baby is in for, here are some notes from our taste test session.

CARROTS

In comparing Gerber's regular and organic carrots (1st Foods), we found that both tasted sweeter than fresh carrots that we cooked in water and then puréed. The commercial version of the regular carrots, in particular, also had a very bitter aftertaste. And while the carrots that we puréed in a food processor were bright orange, those from the jars were darker and much less vivid in color.

SWEET POTATOES

We compared the taste of sweet potatoes that were baked and then puréed with a little water, to Gerber's 1st Foods sweet potatoes.

Again, the Gerber product had a more bitter flavor than did the homemade version and, in fact, didn't really taste like sweet potatoes at all. Color comparison: burnt orange for the homemade, versus almost brownish for the store-bought.

PEAS

Again, peas simply cooked in water and puréed in a food processor or blender, or mashed with a fork, were far superior in appearance and taste to the jarred organic product by Earth's Finest that we sampled. The Earth's Finest peas did not taste like peas at all, but rather a gelatinous mix of unidentifiable vegetables.

GREEN BEANS

If you've ever had canned green beans, then you have an idea of what Earth's Finest (organic) version of this baby food tastes like. There is a distinct metallic aftertaste, very sharp and bitter, and nothing at all like fresh cooked green beans. All I can say is, if this is what children think green beans will taste like, it is no wonder that so many of them resist eating vegetables.

BANANAS

The first thing you'll notice when opening the packet of Gerber 1st Foods bananas is the pungent odor, very sweet, similar to an overly ripened banana. The taste of the product, however, more resembles a pre-packaged vanilla pudding than a mashed-up banana.

Are you getting the picture? Commercial baby foods, handy as they may be, are simply no substitute for fresh foods prepared for Baby at home, at least in terms of flavor. In fact, I'll go so far as to say that they may actually be detrimental to Baby's learning to associate "eating" with "enjoyment." This is important to consider, because at this phase in her young life, Baby is at a concrete point along the continuum of palate development that may influence food choice and acceptance for years to come.

"I'm the one who supposedly did everything right," a mother of a three-year-old girl and a one-year-old baby boy told me. "I ate loads of vegetables when I was pregnant and nursing, even things like collard greens and spinach that I don't normally like. I breastfed them both for a year. My daughter's first solid foods were vegetables. But now she won't touch them, and she has too many other weird eating habits to name." This woman is genuinely puzzled as to why her little girl is such a picky eater, especially since she and her husband both love to cook, eat out, and experiment with new foods and cuisines.

We talked about the situation, trying to come up with ideas that may entice her daughter to try something new. As we were wrapping up our conversation, she made an off-hand comment that she needed to "run by the grocery store to pick up some baby food" for her son. Do you see the irony here? She and her husband eat top-quality foods themselves, yet she expressed surprise when I asked about using store-bought baby food. She had never considered that this could be part of the problem she is now having with her older child. "Of course my daughter ate commercial baby food," she said. "Isn't that what all babies eat?"

"If you only give your baby commercially prepared baby foods, rather than homemade, she may have a harder time transitioning to the adult version of the food when the time comes," Pat Harper added. Pat explained her interesting theory to me this way: "Many of the commercial baby foods do not taste like fresh. There will already be a change in the appearance and consistency of the food when the child goes from eating purées to eating true solids. But if Baby has been eating homemade, puréed fruits and vegetables all along, at least the taste will be familiar."

A coincidence? Maybe. But a pattern I saw more than once in my research for this book. So start early—yes, this early—in insisting on quality products in foods that you introduce to your baby.

Who Is Feeding Our Babies?

"My wife and I always gave our three boys 'real' foods, even from the time that they were babies and were first starting to eat. We had a blender and a food processor and just put everything in one of those to prepare their food."
Chef John Brand, Las Canarias Restaurant, San Antonio,
father of an eleven-year-old, a seven-year-old,
and a three-year-old

The infant food industry in the United States is a big one, worth $1.25 billion a year, primarily to the three major companies (Gerber, Beech-Nut, and Heinz) that control 95% of the market.[32] The other 5% is made up of much smaller, relatively new companies, many of which are trying to take advantage of the growing interest in organic products. If you've recently had a baby, chances are that you've experienced the reach that these companies have, through direct mail pieces, advertising, coupons, and give-aways at your doctor's office. They track down moms and dads in much the same way that the formula companies found you when you were pregnant or first gave birth.

And while much of the information disseminated by these manufacturers is helpful to new parents, be aware that their number one goal, always, is to sell product. To do that, they need to convince you that you are better off relying on their expertise and the convenience that they provide, rather than taking matters into your own hands and doing what may be better for your family. Important factors that they neglect to mention, such as the cost, taste, and quality of their product and even some nutrition concerns, may weigh in favor of you, the parent, choosing to make more homemade baby foods and buy less of theirs.

Take their corporate Web sites. While all are written by qualified dietitians and promote universal guidelines established by the American Academy of Pediatrics, the language that they use and the slant that they put on the facts is definitely from a marketing perspective. Heinz's site, for example, claims that while preparing homemade baby food is nutritious, relatively inexpensive, and allows for variety, the "safe preparation of homemade baby foods takes time, knowledge, and effort." Beech-Nut warns, "Don't leave homemade baby food out at room temperature for more than a few minutes." And "If you are going to make your own baby food, don't include carrots, spinach, beets, turnips, and collard greens. In many places these vegetables may contain too much nitrate, which could make your baby sick. The vegetables used in prepared baby food do not contain high levels of nitrates."

"Oh dear," New Mom may think. "If I try to make food for Junior, I might make him sick! If it's this hard or risky, then perhaps I shouldn't even bother." And another buyer is kept in the fold.

Knowing that moms have been feeding babies with homemade food for a lot longer than any of these companies has been in existence, I researched the position of the American Academy of Pediatrics on the subject of nitrates in foods, the major safety point in which the commercial industry claims to have the upper hand over homemade foods. I also went back to Dr. Sydney Spiesel at Yale's medical school to check on the validity of these Web site statements.

It turns out that AAP's recommendation is that babies *under the age of 3 months* (emphasis mine) not be given these vegetables in a homemade state, as a preventative against the possible presence of nitrates. But, I ask you, how many babies that young are eating any solid foods, let alone these more advanced vegetables? This detail is omitted from the Beech-Nut statement on nitrates. Further, AAP recommends that *all baby foods* (again, emphasis mine) be refrigerated after opening, the homemade and commercial versions alike. In other words, it's no more convenient to take along a jar of commercial baby food that your child may not finish, as opposed to a jar of homemade food, if you're going to be away from home and refrigeration. So it's a matter of how the information is presented that makes the manufacturers' claims a bit suspect.

Dr. Spiesel added that nitrate is "very rarely a problem in foods—I had to search long and hard to find the few reported cases of poisoning in young infants from eating vegetables with excessive nitrates. There are places, as in some swamp regions, that have a soil rich in nitrates, and vegetables grown in those places can have high nitrate levels," says Dr. Spiesel. "This is a very unusual circumstance.

"But nitrates can be a serious problem as a contaminant of well water, and virtually all cases of disease are due to water contaminated with nitrates or nitrites. In infants, this would mean formula prepared with well water that exceeds the approved levels." Aha! So it's formula feeding, not homemade baby vegetables, that is most often the cause of nitrate problems in infants, rare as they are in any case. Is that the message that you would have taken away from these manufacturers' Web sites?

The point is that baby food companies are among the first of many industries that will try to influence you, the parents, in decisions that you will be making on what's best for your child throughout the course of the eighteen-or-so years that he or she is under your control. Any information that they give you will always be from the "product first" perspective. And while that is not necessarily harmful, it is also not necessarily always in your baby's best interest.

A final positive point when considering homemade baby foods is the cost advantage that they offer over purchased products. If you're accustomed to the high cost of formula, then commercial baby foods may not seem that expensive. But even if you're not someone who typically has to think about the cost of food items, take a quick look at these numbers. Then think about how much you'll be spending in the six months or so that Baby would eat these foods, and you can see how much money you would save by going the homemade route.

SWEET POTATOES

Gerber Stage One, organic, 5 ounces	$.31 per ounce
Beech-Nut Stage Two, regular, 4 ounces	$.15 per ounce
Organic brand, Stage One, 2.5 ounces	$.36 per ounce
Homemade, regular, 5 ounces	$.05 per ounce

APPLES

Gerber Stage One, regular, 5 ounces	$.26 per ounce
Gerber Stage One, organic, 5 ounces	$.29 per ounce
Beech-Nut Stage One, regular, 2.5 ounces	$.24 per ounce
Organic brand, Stage One, 2.5 ounces	$.35 per ounce
Organic brand, Stage Two, 4 ounces	$.24 per ounce
Homemade, regular, 5 ounces	$.16 per ounce
Homemade, organic, 5 ounces	$.17 per ounce

BANANAS

Gerber Stage One, regular, 5 ounces	$.25 per ounce
Gerber Stage Two, organic, 5 ounces	$.29 per ounce
Organic brand, Stage One, 2.5 ounces	$.35 per ounce
Homemade, regular, 5 ounces	$.05 per ounce
Homemade, organic, 5 ounces	$.07 per ounce

CARROTS

Gerber Stage Two, organic, 5 ounces	$.29 per ounce
Beech-Nut Stage Two, regular, 4 ounces	$.15 per ounce
Organic brand, Stage One, 2.5 ounces	$.35 per ounce
Organic brand, Stage Two, 4 ounces	$.24 per ounce
Homemade, regular, 5 ounces	$.05 per ounce
Homemade, organic, 5 ounces	$.07 per ounce

PEARS

Gerber Stage One, regular, 5 ounces	$.25 per ounce
Gerber Stage Two, organic, 7 ounces	$.26 per ounce
Beechnut Stage Two, regular, 4 ounces	$.15 per ounce
Organic brand, Stage One, 2.5 ounces	$.35 per ounce
Homemade, regular, 5 ounces	$.12 per ounce

The How-Tos of Making Baby Foods

"Boiling water is the simplest thing you can do, but you do have to pay attention. I'm careful not to over-cook vegetables to the point of them losing flavor. The minute the broccoli turns bright green or the carrots are bright orange, they go into ice water. And then I just purée them."
Sophia, mother of a six-month-old

If I've convinced you of the merits of serving your baby home-made baby food, I hope that I will also provide some relief when I tell you how easy it is to do this. You don't need to be a great chef, subscribe to cooking magazines, watch hours of The Food Network, or even like to cook, for that matter, to make tasty first foods for your child. A pot, a wooden spoon, and a blender or food processor are the only pieces of equipment that I ever used in making Willie or Daniel's baby food, and you can actually get by without any of these. Just substitute "microwave oven" and "mash with fork" to alter these directions to prepare with mini-mal equipment.

Chef Bob Waggoner of Charleston Grill in Charleston, South Carolina, gave me the run-down on the first foods that he used to prepare for his daughter Joyce. "Start with vegetables," he says. "Carrots, zucchini, sugar snap peas, whatever you have available. Take a washed handful and sauté on the stove with a little bit of olive oil. Add a tablespoon or two of water or chicken stock and cook until the vegetables are soft (about 5–7 minutes, depending on what and how much you're cooking). When the veggies are cooked, let them cool a little and then transfer to a blender or food processor. Purée them until smooth, adding more water or chicken stock to get the consistency that you want."

Now what could be easier? It sure beats cooking for adults, right?

One Washington, D.C., chef, the father of toddler twins and another infant, says that he sets aside about an hour a weekend to make his kids' food for the upcoming week. If you're that organized and can block out a little time each week, go ahead and prepare the food, store in plastic sealed containers, and refrigerate until needed. Being a little more scattered than that, I find myself cooking for Baby Daniel every day or two, cooking up whatever vegetables or fruit I happen to have on hand. If I can't find anything fresh, I use frozen; keep a bag of frozen peas, mixed vegetables, or cut-up fruit in the freezer for just such occasions.

There are a few simple food safety rules on baby food preparation to keep in mind. Be sure to wash the fruits and vegetables, just as you would if you were eating them yourself. Vegetables should be well-cooked. And be sure that the food processor or blender, and its blade, are cleaned thoroughly between uses. If you do have some baby food jars from commercial baby foods on hand, run these through the dishwasher before using them for storage of your own foods. Finally, be sure to store all homemade baby foods in the refrigerator, or freeze them for later use.

Infant Mini-Meals

"My kids didn't eat processed, purchased baby foods at all. They began by eating mashed single foods, and quickly progressed to normal people food in small bites and in mashed portions. There's no reason why a 10-month-old can't eat lasagna, for example. I believe that not starting them on processed, jarred baby foods is the number one reason that they don't prefer processed food now. They are remarkably unpicky eaters."
Meredith, mother of a three-year-old and a six-year-old

As soon as your baby is comfortable eating a wide range of foods in their single-ingredient form, you can start mixing things up and giving her what I like to refer to as "mini-meals." Even though these meals may still be puréed or mashed, they can be combined in such a way as to provide Baby with her first taste of real recipes and more complex dishes. These are prepared in the same way that you have been making individual foods; just put the food in a blender or food processor, add a teaspoon or two of water or chicken stock, and purée until smooth.

Include combinations of flavors that mimic real dishes or even menus; for example, tomatoes and chicken; pasta and cheese; fruit and yogurt; vegetables and meat; seafood and rice or potatoes. Make each dish a little mini-meal, all blended together. When preparing a meal or cooking a dish for the rest of the family, get in the habit of putting a few spoonfuls in the blender or food processor, and puréeing to baby's desired texture. Show Baby that certain foods, with their many components such as delicious sauces, are to be eaten together.

And what about the jarred version of mini-meals that you buy at the grocery store? Just for comparison purposes, I sample a few of the commercial "Stage Three" foods, which are generally the first to include meats and vegetables puréed together. Not surprisingly, what you buy at a store has little resemblance in taste to what you can easily make at home:

CHICKEN NOODLE DINNER (STAGE THREE)

Would you believe that the first flavor sensation you get when tasting this is . . . sweet? Must be that pear juice concentrate, which adds four grams of sugar (1 teaspoon) to this six-ounce jar. There is a slight hint of chicken broth as an aftertaste, but no hint of the noodles or carrots that are also a part of this mixture.

VEGETABLE AND CHICKEN DINNER (STAGE THREE)

Ever so slightly thicker in texture than the Chicken Noodle Dinner, but otherwise identical, in color and in taste. This mixture contains potatoes and carrots along with the chicken, but again, these flavors are indiscernible. You can't miss that sweet flavor, though.

From this point, Baby will quickly advance up the food chain, so to speak, eating and sampling more and more adult-like foods. Pay attention to what your pediatrician says about the few foods that should not be a part of an infant's diet until a certain age point (like whole milk and nuts, which most doctors say wait to introduce until the age of one year). Other than those restrictions, he is ready to begin to really enjoy his meals, dining as a real part of the family.

With Baby's food repertoire expanding rapidly, some parents become a bit worried, wondering if they are giving their child food items that are too advanced. Chef Bob Carter of the Peninsula

Grill in Charleston, SC, told me a story about making baby foods for his two sons, Benjamin and Harrison. "I always added chicken stock and a bit of white pepper to flavor fresh vegetables," Carter said. "My wife saw me one day and said, 'You can't do that!' I said, 'Why not?'"

Why not, indeed? As Baby advances in the world of food discovery, it is natural that she will begin to encounter added flavors such as herbs and spices, gravies and sauces, along with foods that offer a range of temperature and texture. As long as these are not hot foods or spicy flavors that will literally burn her mouth or tongue, there is no reason that she shouldn't be trying anything that everyone else is eating.

"You can give them a pepperoni pizza at this point," Dr. Spiesel says.

She's So Sweet!

Bananas, berries, melons, cherries . . . is there a baby who doesn't love the taste of fruit? It's like candy from nature, with a wide variety to choose from, and all good for her, too.

I've included this section on sweets and fruits to clarify confusion that seems to persist on this issue. It's OK for Baby to have lots of whole fruits, right? (Yes.) Does eating a lot of fresh fruit lead to a craving for other sweets, or a preference for other sweet foods? (No.) So, then, that means that other fruity things, such as baby food desserts, fruit-flavored yogurts, and baby snack foods that feature fruits are good, too, right? (No. Stop right there!) This is definitely a case where "sweet" is not "sweet" is not "sweet."

You've probably confirmed with Baby on your own what we know from scientific research: "Sweet" is an innate taste preference, one that we are born with.[33] It's as if Baby's taste buds are attuned to appreciate the goodness of fruit. But there is a big and important difference between the level of sweetness of whole fruits and the sweetness of products that use fruit as an ingredient. In natural, whole form, unprocessed fruits have pulp and fiber, and sometimes acidity, other elements that help offset the sweet taste. You get some sweet flavor, but not a blast of it, as there are other characteristics to the food to balance out the overall profile. Not so with baby food products that feature the fruits in concentrated form.

Take the fruity finger foods of the Gerber and Beech-Nut baby food lines, for example, or their jarred desserts. Gerber offers baby food desserts with sophisticated-sounding names like peach cobbler, tropical fruit medley, vanilla custard pudding with bananas, and Hawaiian delight. From Beech-Nut's "baby bakery" line come banana puffs, strawberry apple puffs, and banana cookies.

The first question I would ask about these products is this: why do babies this age need to be eating "desserts" at all? Most of the jarred baby food fruits are already sweet; why is a special category needed for desserts? How are they different from plain fruits? Is this something that parents buy so that Baby can have a treat at the end of a meal, in the same way that other family members do?

I took those questions to the Gerber consumer hotline, and was told that these dessert products exist "to offer consumers a choice." The desserts do have additional ingredients in them to make them thicker or creamier, to give them more of a dessert-like texture, as opposed to the fruit products, which are supposed to look and taste more natural. The Gerber banana yogurt dessert, for example, contains rice flour, presumably to make it seem more like a parfait, while the peach cobbler contains rice flour and cinnamon to represent the "cobbler" flavor.

But what you need to keep in mind is that these commercial dessert products *taste* super sweet on the tongue; in many cases, even sweeter than a comparable homemade recipe. This is thanks in part to the manufacturing process. To make a peach cobbler into jarred baby food, for example, Gerber uses a peach purée and a white grape juice concentrate. That adds sugar, so much so that the total content in a four-ounce serving (that's one-half of a cup) is 13 grams—just over three teaspoons. So now you have not only puréed, condensed peaches, which taste sweeter than the fresh peaches that you may use if you make real peach cobbler at home, but also a sweetening agent that is added to the mix. The end result? Very, very sweet.

If you don't want your child entering toddlerhood with a sweet tooth already formed, watch the amount of *processed fruit products* you let him eat. Note again that this is *not* the same thing as limiting his consumption of *whole, fresh fruit.* Almost all fruits in their natural form are wonderful foods for older babies.

And for goodness' sake, if appropriate, teach Baby *now* to eat fruit and like it with the skin on. Apples, pears, peaches, plums, nectarines, grapes: all of these have important nutrients as well as fiber in the skin of the fruit. Eating them skin-on also reinforces the important message that whole fruits are better than anything that is in any way further-processed. Start peeling the skin of the apple today, and the next thing you know you may have on your hands a child who insists on them being served this way every time. From there, it's a quick step down to apples that must be red, apples that must be sliced, or apples that are really apple juice or applesauce.

As long as Baby is getting the other nutrients that he needs in his diet, you almost can't give him too many fruits. These fresh foods are the perfect level of sweetness for babies this age. But take them a couple of steps down the processing chain, give Baby too much of the concentrated versions, and you could be setting him up for a long-term craving of a greater intensity of sweetness. Best to stay away from packaged sweet products of any kind at this age, and give sweet Baby her sweet fill exclusively in the form of whole fruit.

Improving Flavor

"I do think it's all about flavor and texture. Green beans with linguine and homemade pesto are a total hit. He won't eat plain chicken, but a pungent satay on the grill kept him busy at a barbeque. And at first he didn't like peas, but then tried an Indian curry dish with peas and cheese and was hooked."
Sonya, mom to a two-year-old

Recently, I was in the midst of a typical rush period, trying to get my boys ready to leave the house for an afternoon event. I wanted baby Daniel, especially, to stay on his schedule as much as possible, so I decided to prepare a quick lunch for the three of us to eat before we left, rather than waiting to eat when we got to wherever we were going. The only thing that I had readily available was leftovers from the meal I had served the night before: a chicken, spinach, rice, and lima bean concoction that I make often for our family. It is flavored with lemon juice and balsamic vinegar and is really quite tasty. The night before, Daniel had eaten it heartily. This particular afternoon, he was having none of it.

After ten or so precious minutes of patiently trying to help Daniel eat, only to have him laugh at my efforts, spit out the food, drop it on the floor, push rice and chicken around on his high-chair tray, and let me know in every other way possible that he didn't want it, I briefly considered an easy out. The simple answer would be to give in and get him something that I knew he would eat, such as pasta and cheese or maybe a bowl of yogurt. But I stopped myself: what message would this send, to Daniel and also to Willie, who was quietly watching every step of this drama unfold? Complain about your food, refuse to eat it, and you'll get something else?

"But he's just a baby, and he has to eat!" I thought, like we've all thought. "Yes, and this is perfectly good food in front of him now," the other side argued back. "You just have to convince him of that."

Willie was picking at it too, and after taking a bite off of my own plate, I realized what the problem could be. While the flavors had intensified overnight, the meat had dried out a little, and the spinach and rice were almost soggy. It really wasn't as good as it had been originally.

So, still on the clock, I took everyone's food back to the kitchen. I put it all back into a saucepan and warmed it again on the stove. While the food was heating, I added some chicken stock, a few drops of balsamic vinegar, a teaspoon of olive oil and a pinch of black pepper. I also spotted a bag of dried cranberries in the pantry. "A new food for Daniel," I realized, and dumped some into the pan.

Before re-serving the dish to Daniel, I showed him some dried cranberries so that he would recognize them cooked with the chicken. He tried a few, and seemed to really like them. Then an interesting thing happened. I put a little of the reheated casserole on a spoon and showed it to him. He immediately went for a bite that contained a small dried cranberry, and then continued eating ravenously until he had finished the entire serving, and then some. He looked closely at each spoonful before eating it, to determine, I suppose, whether or not this would be a cranberry bite. But he was fine either way, with or without. Once the dish was doctored up and the flavor improved all around, even this baby found it much more palatable. Maybe he's farther along on this palate development track than I give him credit for!

Even at a young age, babies respond to flavor, so don't be afraid to spice things up when preparing these meals. Many of us shy away from spices when preparing foods for our littlest ones to eat, but I think you're doing Baby a big favor if you include flavorful additions to her meals. (Of course, this does not mean hot spices; stay away from anything that could burn the tongue!)

If you're nervous about this, start with simple or sweet herbs such as mint and lavender, spices such as cinnamon and ground ginger. Cookbook author Monica Bhide says that her year-old son already likes spicy things, but "I don't add cayenne pepper or red chilies to his food. But I do put in turmeric and coriander, as well as other spices that add aroma and flavor without adding heat." This is a gentle and delicious way to start Baby down the path of appreciating the complexity of various dishes.

So What About Organic? Is It Fresh?

"My daughter just loves ketchup. She wants it on everything, even weird
stuff like fruit. Sometimes I worry that she is getting too much of this,
so I always make sure that at least I'm buying organic ketchup."
Melissa, mom to a twenty-six-month old

"I make 95% of my daughter's food from organic fruits, vegetables,
and rice. For ready-to-eat food, we use organic yogurt and milk. But
yesterday my husband gave her salt and vinegar chips. She didn't
implode and I'm sure the chips won't give her boils. I just try to make
healthy choices with the knowledge that I have."
Posting on parenting Web site

Is it fair to compare apples to apples? That's exactly the question when considering apples that are organically grown, and those that are conventionally grown.

I've read and heard a lot of discussion among moms and others as to whether or not organic foods are the best for our families to eat, as in safer, healthier, and better tasting. There are more organic products available, through more grocery store chains, than ever before. No longer the food choice of the earthy set alone, organic products grew 20% in sales in just the last 10 or 15 years, far faster than most products in the food industry. One quarter of American shoppers buy at least one organic product each week, up from 17% in 2000.[34]

So what is behind all the hype? What is so special about the "organic" label? Why do these foods cost more?

Organic goods are those grown and produced without the use of chemical fertilizers, spray insecticides, growth hormones, herbicides, and the like. Instead, organic farms use crop rotations, natural fertilizers, such as compost and mulch, soil and water conservation techniques, and organic feed for animals. The farming practices are also designed to encourage soil and water conservation and to reduce pollution. All products that carry the USDA organic label must come from farms or manufacturers that are certified as meeting these standards. (An exception is made for producers who sell less than $5,000 worth of food products a year.) If it's a processed product, at least 95% of the ingredients must be organically produced.

Organic foods are more expensive, typically by as much as 10–40%. In a quick price check, I found that Gerber's regular Stage One baby foods sell for about $1.09 per package, and Stage Twos for $1.20 each. This compares to $1.25 for organic Stage Ones and $1.60 for organic Stage Twos. In a comparison of other things that you might buy for your kids, a small container of conventional yogurt was $0.69; a similar-size container of organic yogurt by a different manufacturer was $0.89. In cheeses, I found six-ounce packages of organic string cheese for $4.49 and twelve-ounce packages of nonorganics for $3.59. One-pound tubs of cottage cheese were $4.39 in the organic form and $2.99 in nonorganic. Even if you're not particularly price-conscious when it comes to foods, you can see how this difference can start to add up.

There is some question as to whether or not organic products are nutritionally superior to their nonorganic counterparts. Some organic foods, especially fruits, vegetables, and milk, contain more cancer-fighting antioxidants, says a group of researchers from the United Kingdom, announcing the as-of-yet-unpublished results of a four-year study comparing the nutritional quality of the two.[35] "It's the equivalent of eating an extra portion of fruit and vegetables a day," said Newcastle University professor Carlo Leifert.

Other scientists disagree. "As a botanist, I know that a plant is a plant is a plant," writes UCLA professor Bob Goldberg, PhD, in AgBioWorld. "The structure, cell types, biochemistry, and genetics are the same." Goldberg adds that in some cases, organic produce may be even more risky than conventionally grown fruits and vegetables because organics must rely on manure for fertilizer, introducing potentially harmful bacteria into the process. When it comes to such items as meats, poultry, and dairy products, the levels of fat and dietary cholesterol are the same.

Some say that organic foods taste better than their conventionally-produced counterparts. While that may be true in some cases, I do think that a lot of people make a mistake here in confusing the concepts of "organic" and "fresh," especially when it comes to such things as fruits and vegetables. If something in the produce aisle of your grocery store is labeled "organic," this does not necessarily mean that it is any "fresher," in terms of quality and flavor, than the identical-looking item right next to it that is not organic. For all you know, the organic product is even less "fresh," as you can't be certain how long it has been at the store or what it had to travel through to get there.

The tastiness of such foods as fruits and vegetables, which we often eat raw, is about freshness: *where* it was grown, rather than about *how* it was grown. The closer you are to the source of production, the less distance that the fruit or vegetable has to travel to get to your table, the better it will taste. This is perfectly logical if you think about it. The majority of fruits and vegetables are too delicate to travel well, and, once picked, they start to decompose at a very rapid rate. The strawberries that are grown and picked in California have to travel 3,000 miles to reach a Pennsylvania grocery store. Even in the best-case scenario, it will take several days to get them from the field to the processing plant to the truck to the warehouse to the grocery store to your table. That's too long for a strawberry to exist in top form. Other fruits do travel well, like pineapples from Hawaii. With their tough outer skin, they are up to the journey across the Pacific to the continental United States.

So does this mean that people who live in Pennsylvania and other northern climates should not eat strawberries? This is a tough argument to make in a country whose citizens take in far less than the recommended amount of two cups of fruit and two-and-a-half cups of vegetables each day. If the strawberries are there in the middle of winter, why not eat them? And another related question: what about canned and frozen fruits and vegetables?

If the choice is between eating no fruits and vegetables at all, and eating well-traveled, out-of-season produce, then of course, eating them is the way to go. However, if you want to be a true taste purist, you would wait for the super-tasting local berries to arrive in your area in the spring or early summer. Winter, foodies would say, is not the time to be eating strawberries. Winter is for citrus fruits, such as oranges and grapefruits, which, incidentally, do travel well to and from far-flung locations. And what about your frozen options? Frozen fruits and vegetables are superior in flavor to canned, always, as they usually contain no preservatives or additives, such as sodium or high-fructose corn syrup.

As silly as all of this may sound to some people, I believe that there is an important message here that we can pass on to our kids about the food that they eat and the way that it should taste. There is no question that you will get the best quality in fruits and vegetables when they are local and in season. It's as if nature has given us fresh foods as gifts at certain times of the year, to be enjoyed when the time is right, and to be anticipated and even missed when they are not available. Just because agricultural science has figured out a way to mass-produce those strawberries and fly them around the world year-round does not mean that they have succeeded in getting full-flavored strawberries for you whenever you want them. And if you want your kids to understand what a berry, or anything else for that matter, tastes like in its prime form, why would you want to teach them to be satisfied with a lesser standard?

But back to organics, and whether or not they are worth the added cost, based solely on the taste factor. In determining this "flavor value" of organics, I think you have to put the food products into separate categories: the perishable foods and the non-perishables, the processed foods and the nonprocessed.

It is the perishable foods—fruits and vegetables, milk and cheeses, sometimes meat and poultry—that are generally considered to be superior in flavor in organic form. And in those perishables that you eat raw, such as most dairy products and fruits and many vegetables, you can most readily detect better quality in the organic version. A comprehensive taste test at Washington State University, in fact, found that consumers deemed organic apples to be sweeter than others that were grown conventionally, probably due to the differences in the soil.[36] When I gave Willie a sample of both organic and nonorganic yogurt, he did notice a difference, primarily in their textures, but couldn't decide which of the two he preferred in terms of taste. "They both fill my tummy with yumminess," was his final verdict.

In other foods, the taste difference between organic and nonorganic is not so clear. Cooked products, such as meats and poultry, for example, better reflect flavor imparted by preparation methods than the methods in which they are produced. This is also the case with processed foods, canned vegetables, condiments, pastas, and other packaged goods. In all of these, there was very little, if any, flavor differentiation between the organic and nonorganic versions in my taste-testing.

I'm going to be honest and tell you that I have found very few instances in which I can say that the flavor and taste of an organically produced product *purchased at a grocery store*, compared side by side with the same product produced in conventional form, is really superior, *due to the organic processing alone*. In fact, in most instances, the taste difference between the two is not noticeable. The key words here are *purchased at a grocery store*. In-season produce obtained from your local farmer's market, or grown in your own backyard, will always taste the best, organic or not.

I would not go out and make a big switch to organic foods for your kids solely on the basis of wanting them to have the best-tasting foods. There is simply not enough difference in the flavor to make any noticeable impression. In fact, in the case of the baby foods taste test discussed earlier, the organic products consistently scored the lowest in terms of taste.

If you have health or safety concerns about the mass-produced food that you give your kids, then that is another story, and organic products may be right for you for those reasons.

But when I hear people say that organically produced foods "taste" so much better than nonorganics, I suppress a grin. There is something in the human mindset, I suppose, that wants to believe that we can buy better quality by simply paying more for something. If "better quality" to you means grown without the use of pesticides, fertilizers, and growth hormones, plus the knowledge that you are buying products whose production helped to replenish the earth, then organic foods fill the bill. But in terms of "better quality taste," the name you want is "fresh" or "local," whether the product is organic or not.

What I've Learned

— If you're in tune with your own baby, you'll know when the time is right to start her on solid foods. Don't be surprised if this involves a step backward for every step or two forward.

— Starting Baby on his first solids, such as rice cereal and then puréed foods, is a Big Deal, for both him and for you. Treat it as such. This eating business is an important new skill that will serve him well for the rest of his life. His first tastes of individual foods, such as fruits and vegetables, are priceless.

— There will be messes—oh, will there be messes—as Baby learns to eat. Try, as best as you can, to take it all in stride. She can be washed, her outfit can be washed, the floor can be washed.

— Tell Baby and remind Baby how much he is enjoying his food. Those "yum, yum, yum"s and "isn't this good?"s are so important.

— Give him something new. And then give it to him again, and again, and again.

— There is simply no comparison in the quality of the taste and flavor between commercial baby foods and something fresh and unprocessed that you prepare at home. It's up to you decide what you want your child to taste as he's trying new foods. The green beans from the little jar or packet that you buy at the store do not taste the same as fresh green beans purchased at a market and then puréed in a food processor.

— You can find an endless amount of information about feeding Baby from commercial baby food companies. While some of it may be useful, it is all slanted to portray their products in the best possible light.

— Preparing homemade baby foods and infant mini-meals is some of the simplest cooking you'll ever do.

— Even babies can discern and appreciate well-seasoned, properly flavored foods over those that are not.

— Organic foods, particularly fruits, vegetables, and dairy products, may have a place in your family's diet, but more important to the issue of taste is the freshness factor.

CHAPTER 5

⌘

The Toddler Years: Time to Expand the Palate

"We used to think that my son was a pretty good eater, but I must say that since he's turned two, he's definitely been pickier. For example, he used to love to eat blueberries, but he seems a bit off on those at the moment."
Jude, mother of a two-year-old

He can walk, he can (sort of) talk—and all of a sudden, you have to watch his every move. She's into everything, exploring, climbing, running, falling down, and learning that she can send her parents into a tizzy with the word "NO." (Or, for effect when really wound up, "NO NO NO! I won't do it!") Sweet Baby has sprouted into Independent Toddler, and with this growth will come new eating styles and preferences. It's during these important years—roughly the time

117

between your child's first and third birthdays—that you can lay the groundwork so that a healthy, adventuresome palate can unfold throughout the rest of childhood and even beyond. But watch out; it most likely won't be all smooth-sailing. As luck would have it, this period that is important physiologically in the development of a child's palate is also the time that developmentally, Toddler learns to sprout wings and rebel.

In 2002, University of Tennessee researchers Jean Skinner and Betty Carruth, mentioned in earlier chapters, published the results of an eight-year study that showed that food preferences formed as early as the age of two are often still intact when a child reaches the age of eight.[37] "The strongest predictor of the number of foods liked at the age of eight was the number liked at the age of four," the study concluded. They went on to look at the question of whether or not a toddler's consumption of fruits and vegetables could predict what he would be eating as a young child of six or seven. No surprise here: more studies showed that there is a direct relationship between the amount of fruits and vegetables eaten as a baby or toddler, and the number consumed as a young child. That is reason enough to work with Toddler now, encouraging her to continue exploring a growing food world.

Many people will tell you that this is the time period when their kids who were "good eaters" all of a sudden switched to the dark side. "He used to eat everything," a mom will say. "Then he turned three and the problems started." New York food writer Larissa Phillips told me that her kids both started off with a bang in their eating, but "shut down" at about this age. "My daughter slowly ticked things off of the list of things that she would eat," Phillips said.

Chef Cathal Armstrong, of Alexandria, Virginia's famed Restaurant Eve, remembers some tough times with meals when his now eight-year-old daughter was about to turn three. "She had been a very good eater as an infant, and then all of a sudden, she just stopped," he said. "We struggled with it for a long time. There were nights that there were a lot of tears at the dinner table. The only thing that really worked was patience, not forcing things to make a bigger problem. We found that fighting about food with a toddler is counterproductive. This all lasted about 18 months or so, and has become much better ever since."

In fact, statements of this sort were so common in my interviews for this book that I decided to look into this issue a bit more, to see whether there really is something going on with young toddlers that makes them more resistant to new foods. It turns out that it all falls in line with predicted child development, as well as a little biology.

Anthropologist Elizabeth Cashdan's work at the University of Utah focused on what she refers to as the "sensitive period" for learning about food. From research on rats to sheep to gorillas, it appears that the adage "you can't teach an old dog new tricks" is true; younger animals in all of these cases are more willing to accept new foods than are older ones. This apparently applies to our little humans as well.

Cashdan theorizes that nature provides in young children a brief time period when they are most receptive to new foods. Typically, she adds, environmental circumstances do not change much throughout our lives, so we don't need to continue learning forever which foods are safe and which are not. But having a built-in sensitive period for learning about new foods reduces the risk of harm or death if newly independent Baby ventures forth into risky territory and eats something harmful. And that leads to a reduced interest in trying new things when Toddler becomes, oh, about two or three years old.[38] Interestingly, Cashdan notes, it is houseplants that are the single greatest cause of poisonings in very young children (six to eight months old), an example of how this physiological willingness to root out and try to eat new things that look like food can be carried to a dangerous extreme.

Flavor appreciation and palate development, remember, are ongoing processes. So that means that now, while little one is young and impressionable, is the best time to introduce the spectrum of food flavors, colors, temperatures, and textures, notwithstanding the initial rejections you may receive. Equally important is the message of eating as a social skill, something we do with and for each other. So bring Toddler to the table and pull out a bib (for your child, not you, although that may be tempting too, at times). And have some fun introducing your toddler to the real joys of food.

A Toddler at the Table

"We try, really try, to eat dinner together as a family, but it's really, really hard. With our older kids' school and sports schedules, the baby's naps, and our work and travel schedules, we're lucky if we can pull it off once a week. Often it's either my husband or me and just one or two of the kids, but I do try to have a set dinner time and meal for everyone who is available."
Lyssa, mom of a seven-year-old, a five-year-old,
and a two-year-old

Here's a point that some more practical (sane?) parents may disagree with, but that we have found to be very important to introduce at this time in our children's lives: to the greatest extent possible, Toddler's mealtimes should correspond to those of the rest of the family. This quite likely won't work for every night of the week, but aim to do this as often as you can.

The benefits of eating meals together as a family are well-documented. This is also increasingly hard to achieve with our fast-paced lifestyles, and it may get harder, not easier, to do this as your kids get older and involved in more activities. But that doesn't mean we shouldn't try, as often as possible, to sit down together, however briefly, for family meals, with Toddler secure in her place at the table.

"But we're lucky to have dinner on the table by 8:00 at night!" you might say. Or, "The only peace and quiet my spouse and I get together is over a glass of wine after the kid(s) have gone to bed." Yes, true, I know. But think of it this way: children at this age don't care what time of the day or night they're eating, but they do care that they are with you. (As opposed to your average teenager, who very likely won't appreciate the benefits of daily meals with Mom and Dad.)

If you or your spouse doesn't get home from work until late, try to adjust everyone's schedule so that at least some portion of dinner can be shared together. This is an important and fundamental first step that will serve children well for the rest of their lives. Better to alter your little one's schedule and give her a late afternoon nap and snack so that she can wait to have dinner later, than to feed her separately every night because the rest of the family isn't ready for dinner yet. At the young toddler stage, particularly, children can always sleep later the next morning or take a longer nap the next day. Doctors will tell you that kids this age need about 10–13 hours of sleep a day, and when they get it is not as important as the fact that they do get it, and how they function when awake.

"We'll do this when the kids get older," some rationalize, thinking that it's too hard or too stressful to force toddlers to wait for dinner, sit through dinner, or behave themselves throughout the meal. "Difficult" and "stressful" don't mean that it shouldn't be done, however, and you may find that it is actually much simpler to get children into this routine when they are very young than to wait until their elementary or middle school years, when precedents have been set and homework, friends, and activities will compete for attention.

"I wish I'd started the family dinner sooner, when the kids were even younger," says food television personality and author Sara Moulton, the mother of two grown children. "When (my son) was five and would wriggle around the table, my husband would say, 'I don't think he's ready for this.' And I'd say, 'well, you've got to start somewhere.' So in the beginning, even if he sits there for five or ten minutes, I don't care. At least he's understanding that this is important, and this is something we're going to do."

Anyone with kids will tell you that children at the toddler stage generally do best with a predictable schedule and routine, and that includes time for eating. It may sound confining to think that you always have to produce food at a predetermined hour, but in the long run it makes things easier for everyone when you can anticipate hunger-related meltdowns and prevent them from happening. Getting Toddler on a set schedule for eating is not that difficult, but it does require some discipline and consistency. Think long and hard before allowing Toddler to slip into "he eats when he's hungry, whatever time of day that happens to be" patterns, even for just a few days. In my experience, even a short period of this—such as when we've been on vacation and have let things slide—can result in a more difficult transition back to the norm than you might imagine.

"My son has never been a breakfast eater," a mom of a six-year-old told me. "He might eat a little something, then a snack or a few bites at school, and when I pick him up at 3:00 in the afternoon, he's absolutely famished. So then he wants to start snacking and eating, all afternoon, through dinnertime and until he goes to bed." This mother seemed to think that this is some-how "normal" for her child, as though he's a special breed of kid who, for whatever reason, is programmed to prefer to eat later in the day. She has never considered that he eats this way because she has allowed him to do it for so long.

I think that we're all so used to respecting the bizarre work, hobby, and lifestyle schedules that many adults keep that we for-get that children aren't automatically hardwired to prefer to live a certain way. Babies are not born to be "non-breakfast people," "late-night snackers," "night owls," or any of the descriptors that we so readily ascribe to our friends and relatives. Babies, who grow up to be these eccentric toddlers, follow the schedules that we put them on. If you think it's important for your little ones to eat set meals at more-or-less prescribed times of the day (which it is), and you take the time and assert the discipline to make this happen, then that's what they will learn to do.

All of this adds up to another important point: it's important that Toddler have a sense that eating is something that we stop and take time out to do. Meals have a starting point and an end-ing point. Translation: no eating on the fly or in the car, at least not on a regular basis. Time spent munching while sitting in traf-fic in your SUV does not count as "eating together."

The image of Cheerios and spilled juice all over the backseats of minivans is so well-worn that it's comical. This is actually the age where many people's lifelong habit of eating in the car, grab-bing lunch on the run, and dining to go, begins to take root. But I can promise you this: if you can hold your kids, including Tod-dler, in line on this one (and yourself, by the way), you will all eat healthier and probably better, too. This is another instance where "no exceptions" must become the mantra, unless the situation is so dire (you're stranded in a snowstorm with no gas, for exam-ple), that you truly have no choice but to eat in the car. Most of us would count a toddler meltdown as a dire situation, and you'll just have to judge that one on a case-by-case basis. I think it's a good idea to have a small bag of Cheerios or some other snack on hand just in case, and only *just in case*, of emergency. Being ten minutes from home after swinging through the drive-thru to pick up dinner, and having to resist the temptation to start nibbling on the fries in the bag, does not count as an emergency!

Why is this so important, if you are trying to teach the lessons of "good" foods? What does this have to do with taste?

Because when you eat in the car, or allow your children to, you are stating that everything else that you or they are doing is more important than your time to eat, and what you choose to eat. Wherever you are going or have been is more significant than being at a table, taking the time to taste and enjoy your food. Satisfying your current hunger pangs is more important than recognizing that the hunger is a cue that it is time to stop what you are doing and take care of yourself. The quality and taste of what you eat is not as important as having something cheap and quick (and probably unhealthful) on hand, *now*. Toddlers are all about immediate needs, I know, but as they grow, this is a good way to expose them to the idea that delayed gratification can bring more satisfaction.

For some people, it is very difficult to establish a family routine of eating times. If you're late-night or unscheduled-eating people by necessity, then this is one of the many instances in parenting that you have to do what works best for your family and ignore what everyone else says or does. I have one chef friend who does not get home from his restaurant until around 9:30 every night. His two-year-old is on a schedule that would make many parents cringe, but it works for his family. Most important, his daughter is with her parents for dinner every night, even if it occurs around 10:00 p.m. She sleeps late the next day, but then again, so does Dad.

We can all learn something on this topic from this group of restaurant pros who also happen to be the parents of young kids.

Many of them with whom I talked mentioned the sacrifice of family time that their work requires and the efforts that they make to eat with their kids. Remember, these are people whose hardest part of the work day starts about 5:00 p.m., about the time many little ones at home may be ready for their own dinner. So these working parents have to adapt someone's schedule—their own or their children's—so that they can be together. Many of them say that they have no choice but to turn the day-to-day family cooking over to their spouse.

Chef Robbie Lewis of San Francisco's trendy Bacar tries to slip out in the early evening a few times a week for dinner at home with his kids before heading back to the restaurant in time for the late-night dinner rush. Chef Gayle Pirie and husband John Clark, both chefs and owners of Foreign Cinema in San Francisco, say they have to use a tag-team approach with their nine- and three-year-olds. "One of us is at the restaurant and the other is having dinner with the kids," she says. Many of the chefs make breakfast their big meal of the day with the family; Gary Donlick of Pano's and Paul's in Atlanta tries to cook breakfast each morning with his three-year-old daughter, as does New Orleans' superstar chef John Besh, who says of life with his four sons, "Our big meal of the day is breakfast, and they normally help me with that. They each love to cook different things with me." Bob Carter of Charleston, South Carolina's Peninsula Grill, says that he and his two young sons make up to sixty pancakes at a time on lazy weekend mornings, then freeze them in batches of four for eating later in the week.

If family dinners as a group are out of the question, then try something else. Could the kids have their dinner first, and then a small salad or dessert with Dad when he gets home and is ready for his meal? How about everyone having breakfast together on Saturday, Sunday, or holiday mornings? One weekend day a month reserved for a family lunch out at a special restaurant? Or can Grandma or Grandpa or other extended family members join the kids for some of their meals when Mom and Dad can't be there? At the very least, can the kid's caregiver provide a time and environment where everybody present is eating together at a table or counter?

The point is to establish now a bit of ritual with meals, as well as an expectation that everyone takes part, giving back to as well as receiving from family life. Having little ones at the table sends the message to older kids that everyone in the family has a role to play, we are here for each other, and we make it a point to connect during the day.

Something else that is fun at this stage is teaching Toddler to anticipate the taste of his food. I love to watch Daniel just before dinner time, as he switches on the light inside the oven to see what is cooking, or walks around saying "mmmmmmmmmmmmmmm." As soon as I start calling the troops together, he'll run to his high chair, lift his arms, and say, "Up!" or "Din-Din" with a big smile on his face. Sure, he's probably really hungry and is just trying to urge us along, but this still provides a good opportunity to encourage a healthful appreciation of a meal.

So while you're at it, set down a few rules for family mealtimes. Televisions, computers, Blackberries, cell phones, and all other electronic equipment can be banned from the table at this stage with a simple declaration from Mom or Dad, plus a commitment to follow through. Just remember: it may be Elmo and the Wiggles today, but it's Xboxes tomorrow. None of these should be around to distract from the meal or the interaction that you're trying to create. And that goes for reading at the table, too. At our house, we do make an exception for morning newspapers with breakfast, but that's it. At every other mealtime, there are no books, magazines, or anything else allowed. Even if everyone sits there in silence (rare), there is still some connection with each other that cannot exist if one person's eyes and attention are clearly elsewhere.

Then there is the issue of Toddler and his table manners, an oxymoron if ever there was one. If you hadn't spent much time around young children before having your own, brace yourself for a shock. Virtually every child this age—yes, the child who just a few weeks ago was a docile baby, sweetly beaming from a high chair—will, at some point and to some degree, become a terror at the table. Even yours. Top-of-the-lung shrieks, throwing food, overturning dishes, rubbing messy hands in hair—you get the picture, and it's not a pretty one. Entire meals are ruined, restaurants become madhouses, adult moods are soured, all thanks to the antics of one little Toddler who would rather perform than eat. I'm warning you, it's coming!

The best advice I can give you on this is to know when to throw in the towel. There are times that you simply have to say, "You win." If Toddler is tired or not feeling well, his actions are probably reflecting this, and it's best to just downplay eating in favor of resting anyway. If she's wound up over a new environment or guests at the table, try to coax in a few bites before succombing to the idea that the situation at hand is more enticing than the food. These instances should be the exception and not the rule, however. Slowly, even Toddler should begin to get a grasp of the behavior that's expected of her at the table.

When Daniel's bananas or beans are no longer being eaten and are instead serving as missiles to be lobbed at his brother, I know that it's time to call an end to the meal. I give Daniel a gentle "no no," and immediately remove him from his chair, with hopes that he will soon learn to associate these actions with the end of eating. Loud screams are ignored, never rewarded, especially with food! Banging spoons and dishes or squirming and trying to stand up in the chair has an immediate and consistent consequence—he doesn't get to self-feed anymore, for example, or he comes out of the chair and sits in someone's lap. (As long as that's not perceived as a positive thing!) Don't be afraid to set down rules for behavior at the table and to employ a little discipline to enforce them. The good news is that all of this will improve as Toddler gets older, as long as you start now to teach him what is expected.

Finally, this is also a good time to model to your kids that certain foods are for breakfast, others for lunch or dinner or snacking. Cereal for dinner, for example, may have worked well in pre-child days when Mom and Dad ate a big meal during a business meeting for lunch and only wanted a quick snack at night, but it's not appropriate for dinner at home with kids in the interest of healthy family eating. "Children learn very early that certain foods are served in particular order at meals and that particular social occasions require special foods," writes Leann Birch in her account of children's food-acceptance patterns. "Even two-year-olds can tell you what foods should be served at birthday parties and that dessert comes after the vegetables."[39]

The Menu, Please

"We plan meals and restaurant trips entirely according to our own dietary preferences. That has been our approach from day one. My husband is fond of sushi, for example, so when he's out with her, they often end up at sushi places. I like Indian food and Latin food, so I gravitate toward those restaurants."
Erika, mother of a 28-month-old

"When Brad prepares meals, instead of telling the kids what they're getting, he lets them tell him what they want, creating a lot of extra work for himself!"
From "Behind Closed Doors: Brad and Angelina's Nanny Tells All!" *Star* magazine, June 9, 2008

So what should you be feeding your young Toddler at this meal, as he sits proudly in his high chair, waiting (or screaming) for more food to put in his mouth, or perhaps smear on his face?

Just exactly what you are eating, say many of the experts on the subject, ranging from culinary professionals to health practitioners to child development specialists. Aside from obviously inappropriate products such as alcoholic beverages and any foods that may be an issue because of potential food allergies, at this point in Toddler's young life, he is ready to sample as much full-fledged adult fare as you are ready to give him. And in keeping with Dr. Cashdan's report, as well as many other research findings that demonstrate that there are important windows of time when children are the most receptive to new foods, why not start now introducing as many as you can?

Virtually every expert that I spoke to on the subject—doctors, psychologists, chefs, and just-plain-experienced parents—agreed: if you want to want to raise a child who will love to eat everything, you've got to start setting up that expectation at a very early age. And that means this: what we're having for a meal is what you're having for a meal. No exceptions.

Start now with the idea that there is one menu for the entire family. This is a *dinner*, not a *diner*, although kids are prone to confuse the two! Don't go down the path of allowing a special meal for children of any age, including Toddler. Tell your kids that "this is breakfast or lunch or dinner," and you're going to love it! If it's steak and potatoes night, chop up the meat and mash the potatoes and let Toddler enjoy along with Mom, Dad, and whomever is dining together. Serve the youngest eaters the same sauces, side dishes, salads, and vegetables that everyone else has on their plate, just in smaller portions. If Thai, Mexican, Chinese, or another ethnic take-out food is on the menu, all the better. Talk it up and tell your toddler what she is eating. If a certain food is a little spicy, you might stir a tablespoon of milk or sour cream into Toddler's portion. And be sure to let the food cool thoroughly; he won't want his at the same piping-hot temperature that it may be served to everyone else.

I also think that it's very important, even at this age, to start modeling to kids the concept of *meals*, rather than just individual foods. Have you ever noticed that a lot of young children seem to focus on just one or two items that may be separate components of an entire dinner, rather than seeing, eating, and enjoying the meal as a whole? This is a struggle that many parents will face for years, and the seeds of it are planted in these early-eating years. You prepare meals as a whole, with thought to the individual parts. If you eat out at a restaurant, the chef has chosen items that go together for your plate. Start teaching your kids now that this has an important purpose.

For example, say you're having grilled steak, corn on the cob, green beans, a salad, and potatoes for dinner. This represents what most Western meals are composed of: some meat, a starch, and vegetables. If you add a little red wine sauce to the steak, all the better. Perhaps blue cheese dressing on the salad. All of these flavors work well together without overwhelming one another. This is a classic meal, designed to be eaten together with the greatest benefits in nutrition and taste. Kids need to learn as part of their food and flavor education the thinking behind this. Why wouldn't you also serve rice with this meal? Why is a heavy cheese sauce on the green beans unnecessary? Why do the various colors of the foods—the juicy brown of the steak, the yellow and green of the vegetables and salad, the white of the potatoes, the deep red of the wine sauce—make it look more appetizing?

When it comes to eating this meal, kids will most likely be fine with the steak, and maybe the potatoes, too. The corn and the vegetables could go either way; some children enjoy gnawing that cob, others find it too much work. Some will devour a salad;

others will pick it apart and eat only certain parts of it. The green beans may remain on the plate untouched unless there is a bit of prodding on your part. And prod you should, again to emphasize the concept of the whole meal, rather than just each separate part.

In creating a flavorful meal, you wouldn't want too many sauced dishes, as the textures are too similar and the different flavors would end up competing with each other. You typically wouldn't serve a potato dish, a rice dish, and/or a pasta dish together, because that would be too much starch. A lack of vegetables also throws a meal out of balance, as would too much meat protein. Teach your children to think about and eat their meals in this way.

One question that comes up from time to time: what about desserts? If the rest of the family is having ice cream or a piece of pie after dinner, should Toddler be allowed some, too? Yes, I think so, but in amounts that are appropriate to his age. At eighteen months or younger, he will most likely be happy sitting in your lap during dessert, eating just a crumb or two of cake or getting a few dabs of ice cream. The point is to expose him to the sweets as a fitting end to the meal, but not to overwhelm him with the richness. At two or three, he may be ready for his own very small amount of dessert, served alongside the rest of the family's.

This is one area where I think it is worth paying particular concern to the quality of the food, especially as Toddler gets older. Homemade sweets are always the best, of course, along with full-flavored ice creams and other rich goodies. The key—for everyone in the family, not just Toddler—is to learn to be satisfied with a *small portion* of a very good dessert, rather than eating a lesser-quality product in excess. If you like to bake, great; make up a batch of cookie dough, bake just a few cookies at a time, and freeze the rest of the dough for later use. If you don't know a whisk from a rolling pin, that's fine too. Just make a point to purchase your sweet treats at a bakery or somewhere where you're sure you're getting top quality. Chef Zac Pelaccio of the Fatty Crab and Five Ninth in New York told me that he gives his three-year-old son a small piece of dark, bittersweet chocolate after every meal. The child is learning to appreciate the fine flavor of chocolate in its best form and that a small amount of a good dessert is sufficient.

We've seen that child feeding experts believe that there is a strong correlation between the foods that little kids "like to eat" (meaning, those that they will eat) and the food preferences of their family members. And again, while this may seem obvious, it does have a practical application at the group dinner table: parents should not prejudge or stereotype foods that they "think" toddlers will not want to eat; rather, they should expose them to a wide variety of foods.[40] If Toddler sees you and a sibling or two enjoying the meal, chances are greater that she's going to want to jump right in there and eat it, too.

So as she begins to experience different tastes and textures, now is the time to start talking to Toddler about the concept of flavor. The best message is a simple one: all foods taste "good." Foods have different flavors and you will like some better than others, but each contributes to the overall palate picture. And remember to add that "yum yum" as she's trying something new, and learning to taste and savor. Some examples:

- ◆ "Sweet" is easy and probably won't require much encouragement, so let Toddler begin to discern flavor differences here. Apples are sweet and plums are sweet, but they don't taste alike.

- ◆ "Sour" is a fun one; try oranges or sour grapes. And an amazing number of children this age (Willie and Daniel included) love licking lemons, so there is definitely some kid appeal.

- ♦ "Salty" is peanut butter or a piece of good cheese. Teach Toddler that it is delicious, but a little goes a long way.

- ♦ "Sharp" is dark chocolate, anise, broccoli, or spinach. In proper food context, this flavor is called "bitter." But after some debate, I agreed with husband Paul to eliminate that word from our food discussions and replace it with "sharp," although I admit to a fondness for "bitter," as it perfectly describes so many foods. But that word does have a negative connotation in many settings, so better not to use it, I suppose, in communicating to children about something we want them to like. Interestingly, the Chinese use the expression "to eat bitter" to mean "endure hard times." I'm afraid that a lot of tots concur with that as they eat their vegetables.

- ♦ "Earthy" is mushrooms, soy beans, and balsamic vinegar. It's the wonderful "fifth flavor" that is sometimes referred to as unami. This is the most sophisticated of all the flavors, but is one that even young children can take to very easily.

Here's an example of how all of this might play out in real life: One night, I made a dinner of brown rice, steamed carrots, broiled salmon with a sweet ginger sauce, and sautéed arugula. I was rather proud of myself, as I had pulled together fairly easily a meal that I thought would be both healthful and tasty. Willie is a big fan of salmon, so I knew that would go over well. Steamed carrots and brown rice are staples at our house; he would definitely like those. The wilted arugula, to which I had added a little bit of garlic and a splash or two of the ginger sauce from the salmon, was a bit of a wild card. He likes spinach and most other cooked greens, so I decided to try this, hoping that the "sharpness" of arugula would be a nice complement to the ginger sauce, and would work well with the rest of the meal.

I made a point of assembling the foods on his plate so that the flavors would blend together in the tastiest possible manner. I put the brown rice down first, and the greens right next to that. A piece of salmon went on top of the greens, along with a fairly generous pour of the sweet ginger sauce over all. The carrots, topped with a little bit of chopped mint from our yard, went around the edge of the plate and added some bright color. This would be a little test of my "proper flavors" theory about how kids eat.

I cut up the food for Willie and observed how he went about eating it, waiting to hear his comments, especially about the arugula. In typical child-like fashion, he went first for what was most familiar and what he knew he liked: the carrots. They were gone in 30 seconds. Then he paused a bit over the rest of the plate. "I love salmon," he said, almost hopefully. "Oh, yes, I know," I responded.

"And I'm really, really hungry tonight."

"Well, you've come to the right place!" I said, triumphantly. "Yes, this is very good," Paul added, trying to keep up the pace in feeding it to the baby. "Look how much Daniel likes the salmon and the rice and the carrots and the arugula!"

"But I don't like arugula," came the predictable whine. "You've never had it like this," I answered, just as automatically. "You need to try it." Back and forth we went for the next ten minutes or so, as Willie picked around the arugula to eat the rice and the fish. "May I have some more salmon?" he asked at one point. "Sure, as soon as you've finished everything on your plate," Paul and I responded, practically in unison. Willie looked at us both and sighed. Then he put a huge spoonful of wilted arugula on his spoon and, before I could slow him down, put it all into his mouth at once.

What followed was not pretty: a horrified look, a wail, and a dramatic attempt to remove the food from his mouth before swallowing it. But that should have been expected, I realized, as anyone would have had a similar reaction (if not response) to putting that much of such a bitter (excuse me, "sharp") tasting food into the mouth. "Willie, that was too much; too big of a bite!" I said, desperately trying to figure out how to salvage the situation before he swore off cooked greens for life. "You don't eat that much cooked arugula by itself like that. The flavor is too strong; that's why it's served with all of these other things. Here, let's try this again."

And back at it we went, this time with more rice and salmon added to his plate, cut up and mixed in with the arugula, and all topped with another few drops of sweet ginger sauce. I must have been living right that day, because for whatever reason, he picked up his fork again without a fuss. This time, he had a little rice, a little fish, and a little of those dreaded greens, together in one bite. I hope I never forget the happy, surprised look that I saw on his face as he slowly chewed the food. A few bites later, he was picking up a little speed. "This is really good, Daddy. The arugula has a nice flavor!" was the final comment made as he cleaned his plate.

Daddy?

"But She'll Only Eat . . ."

"We absolutely refuse to cater to our daughter. She is not the center of the universe, or even this household, and our thinking on food—she eats what we eat—flows from that."
Erika (again), mother of 28-month-old

"(My daughter) asks me to make her some eggs for breakfast. So I'll make eggs and bacon. She'll eat the bacon but not the eggs. Then she asks for a waffle instead. Both of my kids are very picky eaters. Before I

cook, I ask them, 'If I make this for you, are you going to eat it? Are you sure?' I'm not going to make a waffle so she can waste that too! Now she is mad and still won't touch her eggs. Does this happen to you? How do you handle it?"
Comment on "How Do I Get My Kids to Eat"
section of popular parenting Web site

I can hear it now (possibly from our Daniel's place at the table); the screeches, the shrieks, and the screams. You're trying to get Toddler to eat his sampling of the chicken parmesan casserole or grilled fish or Caesar salad that everyone else is eating, and it isn't going over well. Maybe it's something he's never had before, and he's giving you looks that seem to say, "What are you trying to do to me?"

One thing about kids this age: you can count on them to let you know when they don't like something, especially when it comes to their food.

Food ruts that persist throughout childhood years often start right here, as Toddler is asked to begin consuming from a broader menu. He rebels, parents panic and give in, and the next thing you know, he's eating the same few foods day after day. The specifics may change—first it's cheese sticks or yogurt, then she moves on to insistence on pasta or a single fruit—but the problem of a too-narrow diet can remain for years. I remember distinctly Willie's first food rRut; it took me by surprise in both speed of development and intensity. He was about two-and-a-half at the time.

"Let's head back to the house for lunch," Paul had said after a busy morning running on the beach and playing in the waves and sand. "We have fresh sweet corn, cantaloupe, and those pretty tomatoes from the farm."

"But I want a *sandwich*!" came the reply, and I knew then that we had a small problem brewing. After just a week or two of giving him a turkey and Swiss cheese sandwich every day for lunch during the busy summer weeks of daily pool and playground visits, Willie, my wonderful eater, had fallen into a food rut.

Why do so many of us find it hard to give our kids widely varied diets? This is a bit of a paradox if you think about it, as we have never had a more wide-ranging selection of foods and food products available as we do today. We have so much food in this country, so many choices when it comes to brands and product types and flavors and cuisines. And yet many of us—most of us, probably—eat basically the same products and foods over and over again. Of the approximately 45,000 items in the average grocery store, the average consumer buys only about 150–250 different things each year, and that includes things that you may buy only once, like a spice or other single ingredient for a particular recipe. We know what we like, we buy what we like, we eat what we like. Of course, this attitude transfers over to our kids.

It is at this point that many parents give in to the "default" foods that they know their children like or will eat. When the crying or worse starts ("NO! I don't like that!" is a phrase that comes to mind), it is most tempting to submissively retreat to the kitchen, pull out a box of macaroni and cheese or a hot dog, and buy everyone a bit of peace. "She has to eat something," we tell ourselves. But is this the smart thing to do, as a long-term strategy?

Trust me on this one: if you want to escort Toddler through this culinary rough spot as quickly as possible, this is the single worst thing that you can do. It takes a lot of stamina and resolve to wait out a child who is determined to flex her independence at the dinner table. But I can give you a ray of encouragement by saying that we have found that the nights invested in this extra bit of discipline pay off in big dividends down the line. We have definitely had nights where Willie was still sitting in his chair an hour or more after the rest of us finished eating, but they are now, thankfully, few and far between. These few unpleasant evenings have been well worth the cost to establish the expectation that he will eat and take pleasure in his meal.

Your setup, the way that you announce what Toddler is having for dinner and tell him—yes, *tell him*—how much he will enjoy it, is very important. So many times, we as parents sabotage our efforts right here, by making those negative comments about the food or leaving open the possibility that our kids won't like it. The power of parental suggestion holds fierce sway with children this age, so by all means, use it to your advantage. Christie, the mother of a year-old baby, gave this good example: "I just returned from spending a week at the beach with several friends who have children ranging in age from three to nine. One friend's children ate just about anything that mom put on the table for them, or at least tried it all without fussing. But my other friend's children wouldn't eat *anything*; they even complained about basic things like spaghetti with meat sauce ('I want *plain* noodles'), and forget about vegetables.

"As the mother of a young child learning to eat, I wanted to understand what drove these differences in eating habits. In my observation, the resistance of the 'bad eaters' was completely driven by the parents. At the dinner table, they hovered around their kids like servants, prefacing every bite with comments like, 'I know this isn't how we make it at home, but . . . ,' or, 'I'll make you noodles if you don't like this, but won't you please just try a bite first?' Even silly things like, 'Are you making a face because you don't like your dinner?' I don't think they even realized they were doing it, but it was clear to me that they were actually setting up their kids to refuse many of the meals.

"I asked the mother of the 'good eaters' about her secret. She said that she's fed her kids whatever she and her husband were eating since they began to eat real food, with no fuss or question or alternative choices. She felt like a big part of getting her children to eat well was simply presenting a positive, upbeat attitude about whatever was being served. It seems to me from watching all of this that a critical component of children's eating habits seems to be the attitude of the parents."

Chef Marc Murphy of New York's popular Landmarc Restaurant puts it this way: "My mother-in-law doesn't eat certain things and I said to her, 'please, don't ever say anything like that around my kids!'" Ouch. Yes, watch it: what you say, what others say, and how you say it, can make all the difference in the world when it comes to kids eating well.

Pay attention to the amount of food that Toddler is given to eat. Depending on what and how many things you're serving, one heaping tablespoon of each item is probably enough. Portion size is important, as it sets up the expectation of what he needs to eat to be healthy and satisfied after a meal. Arrange Toddler's meal in his bowl or on his plate as you would anyone else's food. This sends the subtle message: this is what you need to eat before you leave the table. You can always give him more, if he wants it, but the concept of finishing the meal, no matter how small, is an important one at this age.

People used various words to describe this same practice. The "two bites required" rule is another version of the same theme, as "two bites" is about a toddler-size portion of most foods. "My kids know that they have to take two bites of everything on their plate," one mother of three-year-old twins told me. "If they don't like it after that, they don't have to eat it. Sometimes they don't want more than that, but more often they do, even if they complained about it at first." The "clean plate club" seems to have fallen out of favor as a term, and rightly so, I think, as it connotes forcing a child to scrape down his plate to remove every morsel.

All of this teaches kids an important lesson about the role that they play in society, through this experience in the first community that they know: their family. Not every meal will be a favorite. Sometimes, for the sake of others at the table, we cannot always eat what we want. Other people (like Mom and Dad) have favorites, too. I'm all for letting kids have a little bit of input into meal choices and menus, as long as it is done so in a manner that reinforces family team spirit. "It's Toddler's birthday, what would you like to eat tonight?" "Shall we get pepperoni or sausage on the pizza?" "Who votes for ice cream after the trip to the zoo?" This is *very different* from allowing a young child to voice an opinion on his food day after day, or, even worse, continually asking him "What would *you* like for dinner tonight?"

Child behavioral researchers have looked at this issue from a sort of chicken-and-egg scenario: do we not serve new and unfamiliar foods to kids because they refuse to eat them, or do kids refuse to eat new and unfamiliar foods because they are never served to them? We have seen that it sometimes—oftentimes— takes multiple exposures to a new food before a child will grow to like it. But too often, I think, parents in general, and moms in particular (because they are the ones who do most of the child feeding), just don't make that prolonged attempt.

A Carruth and Skinner 2000 study in the *Journal of the American College of Nutrition* really dissected the long-term causes and effects of food pickiness in toddlers. (Like yours? If it makes you feel any better to know this, I can tell you that there are plenty of other people dealing with these same issues in their kids.)

For starters, it appears that a lot of moms of Picky Eaters who participated in this study had just about given up on trying anything new themselves. It had been an average of over four months since these 71 mothers of toddlers had tried any new food or recipe. Some said that it had been as long as three years. Only 20% said that they actively sought out new recipes and tried them just to be serving something different. This group of moms gave their toddler children an average of fewer than six new food offerings *per year*. Even in restaurants, at day care, and during other away-from-home eating occasions, most of these children ate the same thing that they did at home, rather than using that adventure as an opportunity to taste new foods.[41]

Also interesting from that study: it appears that children who are picky eaters are more likely to be disruptive and exhibit bad behavior (read: scream, yell, cry) at mealtime. This is news, you ask? Probably not if you're living through it every day, but worth keeping in mind is that good conduct at the dinner table and a willingness to eat all or most foods go hand in hand. The best line, however, is that almost all of the moms in this study reported that their kids' table manners, as well as the amount of food that they ate and their willingness to try new foods, was much improved by the time the child turned, oh, about seven years old. See, you don't have that far to go now, do you?

A Carrot or a (Fish) Stick?

"I feel like we've tried everything to get her to eat better. We've bribed with the promise of ice cream if she'll just eat some vegetables, and we've also gone the other route, telling her no dessert for a week if she doesn't eat her peas. Nothing works. It's like she hates the vegetables more than she loves the ice cream."
Cara, mom to a five-year-old

Desperate times call for desperate measures, and many parents say that they are not above using bribery to get their young kids to eat nutritious foods—or punishment for not eating them, to use the same psychology, in reverse. Is this a smart move?

Psychologists have looked at this question from several angles. Because of the traditions in Western cuisines and styles of eating that place sweets at the end of a meal, we have a perfect setup for using desserts as "rewards" for finishing the previous courses. "Finish those vegetables and you can watch TV/read a story/stay up later/have dessert," or whatever "carrot" works particularly well at your house. So what really happens when parents try to get kids to eat foods that they don't want to eat, by making attractive promises? Not necessarily what you're hoping for.

In one study on a preschool class, all of the kids were given two snacks of "equally medium appeal," meaning that they were foods the children liked well enough, but weren't particularly favorites. Some of those children were given the second snack to eat automatically after they ate the first, while the others *had to finish* the first snack before they saw the second. The result? The children who were required to eat one snack to get another decided that they didn't like the first snack at all, but that they really, really, really liked the second snack, which they saw as a reward. The kids who were allowed to eat both snacks in their own good time didn't change their preference level on either snack food at all. So these researchers conclude that the best way to go about this is just to present all foods in the order that they should be eaten, as in "eat your dinner, and then we'll have dessert." Dinner and dessert are presented on equal grounds. The mistake seems to be turning it into "eat your dinner *so that you can have* dessert."[42] It's a subtle nuance, but apparently an important one.

Dr. Leann Birch of Penn State looked at this question, too, as part of her 1995 study on children's food acceptance patterns. Birch and her colleagues also found that the strategy of having a child eat a food that she does not care for in order to obtain a reward only reduces the child's liking of that food even more.[43] It's as though their little minds create an association between that food that they already don't like, and work, or a barrier, to get to something that they do want.

Birch had preschool teachers give 64 children two snacks a day for six weeks. Some of the children were given their snacks as a reward for good behavior, coupled with a lot of praise from the teachers. Others received the snacks in a more neutral form; it was presented in a friendly manner, but with no fanfare. And some of the kids just had snacks left for them on their tables, with nothing said to them at all. At the end of the study, and even for some time afterward, the children who had received the snacks as rewards and accompanied by praise had a significantly increased preference for that snack food. Even the kids in the second group liked the snack food better. But the third group, who had no social or emotional ties to the food as it was presented to them, showed no increased preference at all. Another interesting thing about this, Birch noted, was that the sweetness level of the snacks had nothing to do with the increased preference levels, leading to the possibility that all of this positive reinforcement could be used to "increase preference for foods that are not initially highly preferred but are nutritionally desirable." My gosh, could this really work for vegetables?

If you're going the bribery route to get your kid to eat, tread lightly. It apparently works best when the foods are presented in an overall positive way, rather than taking a "no dessert if you don't eat your green beans" stance. According to these studies, all that would do is make the child dislike the green beans even more. But if you can associate a food that Toddler already likes with something that you want him to do, his liking of the food is enhanced even more and you have a win-win situation. I think of a story that my friend Tania told me about her three-year-old son as a good example of this. After lunch one day, little Winn spotted Tania in the kitchen, opening a package of Oreo cookies. Of course, he immediately asked for one. "Here's a cookie," mom said, realizing she'd been caught with them.

"*Two cookies!*" was Winn's reply.

Sigh. "All right," Tania said, beginning to negotiate. "If I give you two cookies, do you promise to cooperate with me by finishing up your lunch and getting ready for your nap right now?"

Silence. "OK," he finally responded. "One cookie."

Here Come the "Kid-Friendly" Foods

"Hey Mom! Make 'life on the go' easier with Lunchables Jr, a tasty, sensible snack for your active little ones. Each snack is made up of foods your kids already love, including cheese, chicken strips, and more. So say good-bye to countless plastic bags for all their goodies. They're all right here in one convenient package."

From the Lunchables Web site

A phrase that enters many parents' lexicons about this time in their child's life is the term "kid-friendly," as in kid-friendly foods, kid-friendly recipes, kid-friendly meals. "Family-friendly" is another version of this, more typically used to describe restaurants. Both of these terms are code for "oriented toward children, not adults." Depending on your station in life at the time, that may or may not seem appealing.

Many moms and dads are constantly on the hunt for foods and dishes that they think will be accepted by their children, served at establishments that openly welcome the little ones. Press a bit, and you'll find that "kid-friendly" or "family-friendly" can cover a lot of territory. As a restaurant descriptor, it generally implies a place that has casual food with an emphasis on quantity and value over quality, an engaging wait staff, a stash of high chairs, crayons, and coloring books readily available, fast service, an ample "children's menu," and a tolerance for noise and unpredictable behavior. In other words, not the sort of place that adults without kids in tow would typically choose to eat if they were in search of a nice meal.

And "kid-friendly" as it refers to specific items on their menus? Think: pizza, grilled cheese sandwiches, juice, yogurt, ice cream, candy and cookies, chicken tenders or nuggets, sugared cereals, pasta with cheese or tomato sauce, fried seafood; let's see . . . have I left out anything? It's amazing to realize that virtually every restaurant you encounter that offers a kids' menu features these identical items, no matter what type of place it is.

It is at this point that many parents, even those who are so sophisticated in other aspects of their lives, encounter and succumb to this "kid-friendly" zone. I'm not sure whether the children's menus that have become a staple in nearly every restaurant, or the numerous children's food products that have boomed on grocery store shelves in recent years, are the cause or effect of this, but either way, if you're a parent of a child this age, it's impossible to miss this phenomenon.

There is something in the mindset of parents now that equates protecting and prolonging our children's youth and innocence with immersing them in a children's world. Of course, when this applies to entertainment, clothing styles, toys and games, language, and friends, that's a good and proper thing. But somehow this protective thinking has also spilled over into food choice, where products and menus marketed specifically to kids reign.

Why is food so different from clothing or video games? Because these special children's foods and menus that so many of today's kids subsist on are not being given to them for positive reasons, such as superior taste or nutrition, or because they are in some other way better for children. In fact, they are designed to appeal to one's basest desires: convenience over quality, quick-energy sugar over balanced nutrition, high fat and high sodium over real flavor. As a result, most kiddie foods are actually worse in all of these categories than what adults eat. Unlike, say, clothing or songs or videos, where the "children's version" is usually a clean-up-your-act, purified rendition of what you would find in the adult world, most children's food is simply a dumbed-down, artificially-enhanced, flavor-neutral knock-off product, laden with at least one of the Big Three.

Morning Wake-Up Call

"I realized recently that my kids have been eating basically the same cereal almost every day of their lives, for ten, twelve, and fifteen years. It's amazing how inflexible they can be in choices of cereals. I don't get it, because they all taste about the same to me— like sugar-coated corn or oats."
June, mother of three older kids

A good example of a food in which the kid version is typically less healthful than the adult version is breakfast cereals.

Most of us have our favorite, sometimes a lifelong favorite, as brand loyalty can be very intense in the cereal world. Even with concerns about a lack of time for breakfast, and the fact that almost one-fifth of all adults routinely skip breakfast, Americans still consume 2.7 billion boxes, or about 160 bowls per person, each year. Of course, many of us eat cereal throughout the day, as a snack or for another meal, not just in the morning. As much as one-half of all children between four and 18 years of age regularly consume cereal for breakfast.[44]

The United States is the fourth-highest cereal-consuming country in the world, behind Ireland, England, and Australia.[45] We have nearly 200 brands, 20-plus new products a year, and many different kinds of cereal to choose from. Some of these cereals are top-notch in terms of nutrition—high in protein and fiber, fortified with vitamins—and even boast government-approved health claims, such as cholesterol-lowering abilities. And just about all of the cereals that can be called nutritionally sound, wouldn't you know, are those that are marketed to adults, rather than children.

The rise of breakfast cereal in this country has a bit of a storied history. It started out strictly as a health product, during a time after the Civil War when Americans were increasingly interested in their bodies and how to take care of them. The Kellogg brothers of Battle Creek, Michigan, came up with the concepts for granola, wheat flakes, shredded wheat, and corn flakes, partly as a result of their work at the Battle Creek Sanitarium. Charles W. Post, a one-time patient there, developed Grape-Nuts. Thanks to some of the first national advertising campaigns, Kellogg and Post were both running successful companies by the turn of the century.

In 1937, Minnesota-based General Mills developed a puffing machine to use on cereal pieces and came out with Kix, the first puffed cereal. The same puffing technique was later used to create "Cheerioats." With the boom of babies at the end of World War II, a new cereal consumer was born: children. To appeal to them, cereal manufacturers sweetened up their existing product base and came out with new, just-for-the-kids brands. Sugar Smacks was one of the first in 1953; at that time, 56% of that product was sugar.

To advertise to kids, cartoon characters must be involved, and these came out in force throughout the 1950s and 1960s to support the burgeoning market for kiddie cereals. The first mascots were the Rice Krispies elves, followed by Tony the Tiger and the Trix rabbit, who soon had children across America chanting "Silly rabbit, Trix are for kids!" (How perfect is that?) Most of the cereal characters popular 30 or 40 years ago are still around today, leading adults to buy these cereals for their own kids and grandkids (or themselves) out of a sense of nostalgia.

As kids' tastes and these cereals have evolved through the years, their packaging and advertising have also progressed with the times. So, too, have the very names of some of the products. Remember eating Sugar Smacks or Sugar Pops as a kid? Overt use of the word "sugar" is now verboten in the children's cereal world, which is interesting, considering that it is still a major ingredient in the products. These are now known by the slightly healthier sounding monikers Honey Smacks and Corn Pops. Frosted Flakes were Sugar Frosted Flakes until the 1970s.

As our taste preferences grow up, some of us move on to adult cereals, many of which are just as high in sugar content as are these kids' products. But there is a difference: in most of the adult products, the high sugar content can be attributed at least in part to the raisins, apricots, or other dried fruits that are a part of many of the cereals. For example, if you like Basic Four cereal, you are consuming 13 grams of sugar with every cupful. But about one-fourth of that is natural sugar from the raisins, dried cranberries, dried apples, and dried prunes. And while it tastes sweet and reacts similarly in your body as added sugar (sucrose) would, you are at least getting the benefit of the nutrients and the variation in flavor provided by these bits of dried fruit.

Fruit does not make an appearance in your child's bowl of Apple Jacks, Froot Loops, or Cocoa Puffs. There, the sugar content (13 grams, 13 grams, and 12 grams, respectively) is made up entirely of the pure white stuff. Presumably, this added refined sugar is there to make the taste of the cereal "acceptable" to young children.

The cereal the parents are eating themselves "is probably better [nutritionally] than what they're feeding their child," says Dr. Marlene Schwartz, a psychologist at Yale University, who recently completed a study looking at 161 different cereal brands. "The majority of children's cereals in our study, 66%, failed to meet national nutritional standards, mainly because of their high sugar content. Overall, there were important differences in nutritional quality between children's cereals and non-children's cereals."

Take Cheerios, the best-selling of all cereal brands. There are several versions of this popular cereal, starting with the original, which is promoted to older adults who are interested in the cholesterol-lowering properties of the oats, as well as for infants, who consume it as a first finger food. With just one gram of sugar and three grams of fiber per serving, plus whole-grain oats, Cheerios is an excellent cereal choice for just about everyone.

Then there is Multi-Grain Cheerios, also for the adult market, and Fruity Cheerios and Apple Cinnamon Cheerios for the post-finger-food set. All start as the same basic, round oat product and have enhancements designed to appeal to the target consumer. Multi-Grain Cheerios, made of corn, oats, barley, and rice, has 110 calories in a one-cup serving, along with 6 grams of sugar and 3 grams of fiber. Not bad, and tasty to boot.

But what happens when you move, or rather your kids move, to the Fruity Cheerios or the Apple Cinnamon Cheerios? Sugar and caloric content go up, fiber content goes down. The kiddie versions are basically the same product, but with corn syrup, brown sugar, orange juice concentrate, and/or apple puree concentrate added as additional sweeteners.

It had been years since I had eaten any of these kid-oriented cereals, so I went out and bought a wide variety and lined up the bowls, spoons, and pitchers of milk. It was time for another taste test!

Here are some notes from my observations about the taste and content of popular kid's brands.

KELLOGG'S PRODUCTS

Apple Jacks
Cinnamon and apple (primarily cinnamon) are still the predominant flavors of this cereal that you probably remember from your own childhood. The "A is for Apple, J is for Jacks" jingle was one

of Kellogg's most popular. It's still a very sweet cereal, providing 13 grams of sugar per serving. Apple juice concentrate and non-visible dried apples are listed as ingredients.

Cocoa Krispies
The chocolate version of Rice Krispies, this is truly one of the sweetest cereals around. These little bitty cereal pieces have 18 grams of sugar in a one-cup serving. Take in a spoonful and you get hit with chocolate; not surprising, since both cocoa and semi-sweet chocolate are major ingredients.

Corn Pops
Once known as Sugar Pops, these puffy cereal pieces taste slightly like corn and a lot like sugar. There is also a new Chocolate Peanut Butter Pops that I did not sample. Sugar content is 12 grams in less than a cupful of cereal; slightly less in the chocolate peanut butter version.

Froot Loops
The real question: do the many different colors of the Froot Loop pieces have anything to do with the flavor? Shouldn't the red pieces taste a little like strawberries, the blue ones like blueberries, the yellow, green, and orange like citrus fruits? Maybe they should, but they don't, at least not much. At one point, I thought there was a slightly lemony tang to a yellow piece of cereal, but that was only after reading the ingredients panel and noting that natural fruit flavors are an added ingredient. Mostly, this Toucan Sam cereal tastes like sugar, which is primarily what it is. You get 13 grams in less than a cupful.

Frosted Flakes
Since 1952, when Kellogg's started coating their flagship product Corn Flakes with sugar, Tony the Tiger has been telling kids that Frosted Flakes are Grr-reat! These, too, taste just as you may remem-

ber them: a bolt of sugar first, with a little bit of corn flake on the side, with 13 grams of sugar in a one-cup serving.

Honey Smacks
If you ate Sugar Smacks as a child, then you know this one. This cereal tastes a lot like it looks, or maybe I just remember it well: the caramel coating is the predominant flavor of the small, puffed cereal pieces that look like tiny hot dog buns. Honey Smacks has 17 grams of sugar (4.25 teaspoons) in a one-cup serving. Kellogg's briefly tried to replace the familiar mascot, Dig 'em the Frog, with a more honey-friendly bear, but consumers didn't approve.

GENERAL MILLS PRODUCTS

Cocoa Puffs
This cereal is basically the chocolate-flavored version of the original puff cereal, Kix. And although the chocolate's definitely there, this cereal didn't taste as chocolatey as did the Kellogg's Cocoa Krispies. The puff shape makes the chocolate a little less intense, perhaps, and you can also make out the corn flavor from which the cereal is made. One cup has 14 grams of sugar. Cocoa is listed as an ingredient.

Cookie Crisps
"Chocolate chip cookies with milk" for breakfast is the idea behind this product, whose cereal pieces actually look like cookies and contain chocolate-flavored chips. There are Double Chocolate and Peanut Chocolate versions as well. Tastes remarkably like store-bought chocolate chip cookies; you just add the milk for the complete effect. There are 11 grams of sugar in three-fourths of a cup.

Frosted Cheerios
If Cheerios are good, then Frosted Cheerios must be better, right? Well, certainly not from a nutrition point of view; the

new version features 13 grams of sugar per serving, compared to just 1 gram in regular Cheerios. With no distinctive cartoon mascot affiliated with the product, this cereal could be considered as a product for adults who like super-sweet, rather than for kids.

Lucky Charms

If you like to eat marshmallows, you'll love Lucky Charms, the colorful cereal that is actually made out of this confection. This cereal has as sweet a flavor as any other kid's product, but the distinctive marshmallow effect is definitely palpable. There are 14 grams of sugar in a one-cup serving size.

Trix

Another puff cereal, this one shaped like pellet balls in an array of pretty colors, brighter than what you find in Froot Loops. In reality, these competing products are very similar and, except for the shapes, are practically indistinguishable in flavor. Both taste a lot like a tutti-frutti candy. There are 12 grams of sugar.

QUAKER OATS PRODUCTS

Cap'n Crunch

Cap'n Crunch now comes in three varieties: the traditional corn-flavored puff cereal, and puffs with peanut butter and "berries" added. Except the berries aren't really berries; this must refer to the multi-colors of the cereals in this box. The peanut butter flavor is the lowest in sugar at 9 grams per three-quarter-cup serving. Perhaps this is because, with the peanuts added, they can get away with a little less sugar in this variety. The berry flavor and the original both have 12 grams of sugar per three-quarter-cup serving.

POST CEREAL PRODUCTS

Cocoa Pebbles and *Fruity Pebbles*
The Flintstones have been the mascots for these cereals since their introduction in 1971, and through the years, various colors and flavors have been added to the colorful Fruity version of the puff cereals. They both taste remarkably like their competition in the "chocolate" and "fruit" flavor cereal categories, and contain 11 grams of sugar in each three-quarter-cup serving.

So, bottom line: what is the result of all this excessive consumption of high-sugar cereals? I didn't find any studies or anyone who could draw a straight line between the consumption of children's cereal and weight or nutrition problems, and any evidence that this affects palate development is anecdotal. Researchers at Monell weren't aware of studies looking at sugar and palate influence in this regard, but they have done similar work on salty tastes. A 1982 study conducted there showed that we become accustomed to certain levels of salt in foods, and really notice when a lower-sodium version is substituted. Most important, we can actually grow to prefer less salt in our food by simply reducing the amount that we use.[46]

So it makes sense to think that this could be the case for sugar and sweet, as well. If high-sugar foods are eaten for breakfast every morning, soon the expectation will be that the morning repast must be "sweet." PopTarts, doughnuts, pastries, soda, and other low-nutrition items eventually fit right in. And maybe this intense level of sweetness also tricks the brain and the tongue into wanting more sweet flavors throughout the day, possibly influencing the choice of food items for lunch or snacks.

Breakfast is still the most important meal of the day. (You do remember your mom telling you that, right?) This applies to you as well as your kids, so as hard as it is, it's worth incorporating the time to eat breakfast into the morning routine. Young children in daycare may have breakfast there; older ones heading to pre-school and beyond also need to make sure that they are eating something either at home or at school before they get too far into their day. But too many of us, adults and kids alike, start the day with "dessert for breakfast," meaning that we eat foods that are high in sugar and refined carbohydrates, and low in fiber and protein. Cereal manufacturers say that cereals are pre-sweetened for consumer convenience. They know that many people, including kids, like to add sugar to their bowls of cereal.

Also, a point about cereal flavors. The last ten to fifteen years have seen the introduction of numerous kids' cereals with an added chocolate flavor. Cocoa Krispies were introduced in 1958, but they have been joined by Chocolate Cap'n Crunch, Reese's Puffs, Cocoa Pebbles, chocolate this, chocolate that. Several chefs that I talked to in research for this book mentioned this trend; one even lamented it as the "beginning of the end" of teaching children about flavorful eating. Why? Flavor confusion, more of that "you can have any flavor you want anytime you want it, as long as you don't care about the quality" idea.

Chocolate is a flavor traditionally associated with after-meal desserts and snacking. It is not what we typically think of as a breakfast flavor to be eaten in the morning, except perhaps as part of a rich beverage like hot cocoa or milk. Injecting chocolate into the morning routine as an add-on to rice or corn cereal dilutes its very value as a candy or baked good. A "chocoholic" you may be, or may be breeding, but doesn't it make sense to teach your kids that delicious chocolate should be enjoyed for what it is, in its own best and proper place, rather than as a mis-placed additive to a sweetened cereal?

Get in the habit of reading the nutrition label on any cereals that you buy, for yourself or for your kids. Check especially for the sugar content; the level will probably surprise you. Fifteen or more grams of sugar per serving is quite common. (For translation purposes, there are 4 grams of sugar in a teaspoon. So that means that 15 grams of sugar is the equivalent of 3.75 teaspoons of sugar.) Kiddie cereals are almost always the highest in sugar content. And remember that the sugar content listed refers to the amount in one serving of the cereal, which is usually one cupful or less—and I bet your kids can eat more than one cup at a time!

If you find this information to be convincing, make yourself a promise that you won't buy or serve a "children's cereal" to your kids. It's best to not let them get started on super-sweet cereals, lest they learn to believe that cereals "should" be sweet. If it's too late for prevention because your children are already used to these products, tell them that a new day has come and that from now on, they will be enjoying other cereals, as in adult-oriented cereals, in the future.

Psychologist Marlene Schwartz says the key is to be adamant about it and not to give in about buying the sugary cereals, not even once. "My advice to parents of young children is you've got to just make a decision and stick with it because if you give in once, you're going to regret it. It's just going to make your kid nag you even more."

"Easier said than done," gruffs husband Paul, and that is definitely true. It may take some gradual phasing out of these super-sweet cereals from the diet, rather than going cold turkey. The Monell researchers found that if people who like high salt levels in their food purposefully eat a lower-salt diet for six weeks, then they come to actually prefer less salt. Might the same be true for the level of sweetness in the diet, specifically with regard to breakfast cereals? As someone who used to eat a 19-grams-of-sugar bowl of Raisin Bran every day and now prefers Grape-Nuts (4 grams of sugar), I personally think so.

You might start by giving your kids a blend of cereals: one or two that contain less sugar, with a little bit of the high-test sprinkled in. We toss a tablespoon or so of gingered granola on the top of a low-sugar, high-grain cereal for a touch of sweetness and added flavor. Willie likes to do this, and refers to the addition as "topping." He is learning to tell the difference in the sweeter varieties and that they are best used sparingly.

Cute, Cute, Cute

"My kids love the fact that a lot of restaurants seem to be all about them. These places go out of their way to really appeal to childlike tastes and appetites. I'm not really sure why, because it certainly doesn't do anything for me as an adult. Sometimes we give in and go where they (the kids) want to go, but I never really look forward to those dinners out. It's like I've signed up for a night in kidville."
Sherrie, mother of a four-year-old and a six-year-old

"Today's kids are exposed to lots of vibrant colors and animation, and they expect these same experiences at the dinner table."
Grocery Manufacturers Association spokesperson, in press release commenting on release of "green ketchup"

Another aspect of "kid-friendliness" in the food world is the many products and family-oriented restaurants that go out of their way to make food and dining appear Fun! Fun! Fun! for children. Am I the only parent who finds this a bit annoying? And not because it's been such a long time since I was a kid myself, but because all of this runs so counter to what I'm trying to teach my boys about food.

Take your average chain restaurant. A lot of parents rely on these places as safe havens to eat out with their young children:

the food is relatively inexpensive, you know what you're getting, and you can be pretty sure that yours won't be the only kids making a scene if something goes amiss. The suits in the chains' marketing departments know this, and they do all they can to make the establishments places of entertainment for the kids. Happy kids equal happy parents, or so the theory goes. The quality of the food is of lesser concern.

And so we are presented with meals and eating situations that are meant to be an "experience" for children. The problem is, that experience has little to do with learning about a new cuisine or proper restaurant behavior, and everything to do with getting another dose of the toys, cartoon characters, and typical food items that some kids eat every single day.

A good example is what I found during a recent trip to a Denny's restaurant. "America's leading family dining chain" has 1,500 outlets across the United States and abroad. One of their recent come-on-in-kids approaches starts with an "outer space theme," featuring "fun foods" like "moon and stars nuggets," "astro dogs," and "flying saucer pizza." "Little astronauts" can also get healthy sides of "anti-gravity grapes" and "far-out fruit medleys." This "galaxy full of fun" promises "lots of activities at the table to keep the kids entertained," and your tots can "choose from rocket cups that turn their drinks blue, green, or red." The children's menu also features some nutrition and exercise tips, right next to colorful pictures of desserts like the "neutron brownie" and "Oreo blast-off."

"But old crumbs like you are not the intended audience," some may say, and believe me, I know that. And I am not saying that your average three- or four-year-old, for whom this show is intended, would not like it. What I am saying is, how could he focus on his food, or attempt to try something a little different to eat, with all of this "entertainment" going on at the table? So as the paying member of the party, who hopes to raise my kids' expectations when it comes to restaurant selection, I have no choice but to make my voice heard by not venturing into this establishment at all.

There are plenty of other examples in the chain restaurant world. Dave and Buster's and Chuck E. Cheese are like giant amusement parks and offer "eat and play" deals where you get a game card with your meal. At Rainforest Cafe, your "dining safari" includes a simulated thunderstorm every thirty minutes, featuring automatic water sprinklers and synchronized lights set in patterns. Hard Rock Cafes are a visual (and aural) shrine to the popular music industry. Perhaps the originator of this tactic, McDonald's is still the best-known, securing its place in children's restaurant lore with Happy Meals, a clown mascot, and playgrounds on many properties.

And of course, there are numerous retail food products that fit into the cutesy category as well. Home-baked chicken nuggets and strips are not simply nuggets and strips anymore; you can find them in the shape of dinosaurs, basketballs, pandas, bugs, stars, and more. Remember having round SpaghettiOs or Alphabetti Spaghetti as a kid? Well, now they also look like cartoon characters or other "fun shapes." Eggo makes "jungle animal pancakes;" Heinz made a splash awhile back with "Funky Purple" and "Blastin' Green" ketchups. Danimals yogurts are all about animals, and each-one-sillier-than-the-next names of flavors. Apple Jacks now sells "cereal straws" to make drinking milk more "fun."

Did I say there is a barrier between the kiddie and adult food worlds? How about a gulf! All of this cuteness is largely what delineates the "child" and "adult" food markets in the first place. Great, if you're a restaurant chain operator or a food manufacturer who wants to segment a market and appeal to its underdeveloped sense of good eating. Not so good if you're a parent of one or two members of this target market, who is trying to help your offspring learn a little about food, and develop more discerning tastes.

And while I'm on this subject, a word about another "cute food" practice that I discourage. Many children's food cookbooks, recipes for kid's dishes in parenting magazines, and mom-oriented television shows and Web sites offer ideas for what they call the creative presentation of foods. These include silly things like making smiley faces out of raisins and carrot sticks or string cheese, or cutting sandwiches into animal shapes and "decorating" them with colorful fruits or vegetables. The theory behind this is that if we turn food into an art project, and make it cute enough, kids will be happy and will want to eat more.

While you may get a few laughs from making a monkey face out of a round of pineapple, black olives and a piece of red pepper, in the long-term, I think that stunts like this send this same bad message to kids about their food: food is not a toy. It is not something to be played with. Even young children can be brought to an understanding that food—good food—is to be eaten, savored, and enjoyed with the senses of taste and smell, as opposed to being used for amusement purposes. We all love to bring out the sprinkles and icing and decorate gingerbread cookies during the holidays, as part of a festive celebration. I do this with my boys and look forward to it every year. But as a daily practice, it does children a disservice to teach that foods need to be elaborately enhanced, or brightly colored, or served up with a side of "fun" to be satisfying.

What Else Is on the Pantry Shelves?

"Raisins are preferred as a snack over grapes, as they are easier to eat and store, and we can be certain that most of the children will like them."
Snack-food guideline in kindergarten parent handbook

As little Toddler begins to expand his food repertoire, you need look no further than your pantry or refrigerator shelves to find an assortment of new foods for him to try. A lot of the products that you may already be buying and stocking up on can be real taste treats. But as you begin to branch out on his food selections, keep this in mind: a *lot* of the processed, prepackaged foods on the grocery shelves have surprisingly high levels of one or more of the Big Three, most likely sodium or sugar. As a result of the processing, or to maintain their shelf life, many of these seemingly perfect toddler foods have a lot of preservatives and sweeteners. And while they do offer some nutritional benefits, most are not the best snack or food choices for Toddler, at least not on a regular basis.

Take applesauce, for example. This staple in many toddlers' diets is sold in handy little one-cup servings that makes it portable and easy to measure the amount eaten. And while the apples certainly make it a nutritious food, keep in mind that some of these products have as much as 22 grams of sugar (five and a half teaspoons) in this one-cup serving. Others have less; Mott's Scooby-Doo Applesauce has 15 grams of sugar per serving, which is about the same amount as in one whole apple. So what's the difference? Why is it better to give Toddler pieces of a whole apple to learn to chew, rather than just keeping him happy with the applesauce?

It goes back to the fact that applesauce is a processed product, making it less-than-ideal in terms of both nutrition and flavor, when compared to the real thing—an apple. A whole apple has pulp fiber, skin, and other elements that moderate the sweet taste. It has crunch and a more complex mouth feel. Applesauce has . . . a sweet taste. Try the two side-by-side and you'll see what I mean.

Raisins and grapes are a similar story. One serving of Sun-Maid raisins, just one-fourth of a cup, or a large handful of raisins, contains a whopping 29 grams of sugar. Raisins are often touted as a good snack, and they are, as they have some iron and fiber and there are only 130 calories in that fourth of a cup. But, still, that's a lot of sugar, and a very sweet flavor. Concord grapes, on the other hand, sport only 15 grams of sugar in a one-cup serving, and just 62 calories. So besides the grape skins, what does Toddler get in a whole grape that she does not taste in a raisin? A bit of a tart flavor and a crispiness from the fruit, to balance out the natural sugar. Once again, the natural and unprocessed version of the grape is the best.

Along with sugar, the other big palate offenders at this point are prepackaged and canned foods that contain added sodium. To a point, they are fine and can be a convenient way to teach Toddler about new foods. But I have found that, in the same way that too much sweetness from processed foods can lead to an adamant preference for sugars, so too can excessive consumption of sodium result in an insistence on salty foods. The problem with both of these, again, is that sweet and salty become the dominant flavors of the food, throwing the whole flavor profile out of balance.

America's kids are well on their way to becoming tomorrow's adults who have serious health problems because of too much sodium in the diet. Remember that the Dietary Guidelines say that children age 2 to 3 should get no more than 1,000 milligrams of sodium each day, and at age 4 to 8, no more than 1,200 milligrams. By age 7 to 9, 68% of kids are consuming too much. "A taste for salt is an acquired taste," says David Jones, president of the American Heart Association. "And kids who eat salty diets grow up to be adults who eat salty diets."

Here are some other examples of common pantry staples that Toddler may like, but should play a limited role in her diet, for that very reason.

♦ Canned baked beans: there are some really tasty ones out there, with flavors such as barbeque, country style, and added bacon. Throw in cut-up hot dogs and you have "beans and franks," a dish many little kids grow to love. Just don't let them love it too much; all of these canned beans are extremely high in sodium, ranging from about 350 milligrams per half-cup serving to more than twice that amount. (And that's without the hot dogs.) A much better choice: make your own using a package of whole beans, which will drastically reduce the sodium content and over-salted flavor. And before you can say "I don't have time to do that," let me just add that this is one of those things that is unbelievably easy to make, as you can be doing anything you want to during most of the prep time. Rinse, soak, and boil. Just be sure to allow enough time for all of the steps; the soaking can be done in as little as an hour (or up to overnight), and some types of beans will cook in 30 minutes. I often start beans soaking in the morning or early afternoon so they'll be ready to cook for dinner.

◆ Pickles: toddler may initially pucker up a bit, but will probably grow to like these, maybe chopped up and mixed in with another food. Jarred pickles are actually a nice little condiment for Toddler, as they are a good way to introduce the concept of "sour." But don't go overboard, and don't let them turn into everyday snacks, as they, too, contain a large amount of the salty stuff. A serving of a leading brand (which is only three-fourths of the entire spear, by the way, not the whole thing), has 710 milligrams of sodium.

◆ Vienna sausages: a perfect size for Toddler's lunch, these make a good first finger food. Just keep in mind: 85 milligrams of sodium per sausage. If you go for the flavored varieties, such as chicken Vienna sausages, it's even more: 136 milligrams per sausage piece. A lot of the flavor comes from the salt.

- Deviled ham spread: same thing—while there is a distinct "ham" flavor in this meat spread, a lot of the taste comes from the 480 or so milligrams of salt in each one-fourth-cup size serving.

- Vegetable dips: dips served with crackers, pita, or small vegetable pieces can teach Toddler a lot about self-feeding, not to mention help her with eye-to-hand control! Just keep in mind that a serving size of dip is just two tablespoons; a lot less than even young children typically eat at one time. And depending on the kind of dip you're talking about, you're looking at about 135 to 150 milligrams of sodium in those two tablespoons. Again, a lot of the tasty flavor is just salt.

- Bottled pasta sauce: so handy to heat and serve over pasta, so many of the many brands and flavors of bottled pasta and pesto sauces are really quite tasty. It's no wonder that many, many moms say they keep these in the pantry to use to pull together a quick meal. But here's the problem: just one-half of a cup contains over 500 milligrams of sodium, about half the amount that a toddler should take in all day.

And there are more hidden surprises when it comes to levels of sweetness.

- Trail mix bars: these popular snack foods are preferred by many parents over chocolate bars, as they do provide some healthful ingredients, such as dried fruits, nuts, or oats. But beware: they are also very high in sugar—about 14 grams per single bar is common. Some of that sugar content, of course, is from the dried fruit, but much of it is added sweeteners. Same result, though: a relatively healthful but sweet-tasting snack food.

♦ Jello and Jello Pudding: quick desserts favored by many in the toddler set, gelatins and pudding mixes are loaded with sugar or, if the "sugar-free" variety, with artificial sweeteners such as aspartame. These products are also surprisingly high in sodium: 18 or 19 grams of sugar (almost five teaspoons) in a half-cup serving size of pudding is common, with an end result, of course, being a dessert that tastes very sweet. And although the flavored regular gelatin does not taste as sweet as the pudding, it actually has about the same amount of added sugar. So don't be fooled; the gelatin desserts have added acids to make them taste more tart than sweet, but the sugar is still there.

♦ Yogurt: there's no disputing that most yogurts have a sweet flavor, whether it comes from natural sugar (lactose, in whole milk), added fruits, or added sweeteners. The sugar content can range from about 12 grams in a four-ounce serving, to about 18 grams or 25 grams, or even more, in a six- to eight-ounce portion. Don't fall into the trap of thinking that low-fat or nonfat yogurt is the answer; these varieties may be lower in fat, but are sweetened with artificial products such as aspartame. More important than fat content is the flavor of the yogurt, and what's added to the product to achieve that flavor. If your toddler loves the stuff, start her off with a plain version (low-fat, nonfat, or even whole) with no added sugar, artificial sweeteners, or flavorings such as fruits. Vary the taste by adding whatever cut-up fresh fruit she prefers, or some nuts or lightly sweetened granola or whole-grain cereal for crunch and fiber.

So you see, Mom and Dad, the products that you may have stored on your pantry shelf can be stored there for a reason: they are usually packed with preservatives that keep them around for a long time. Unfortunately, that preservative, sodium, can immediately go to the top of Toddler's flavor preferences, and show itself again and again as he gravitates toward high-salt foods. And the manufacturing process for other typical toddler foods concentrates the natural sugar so much that the result is a flavor that is even sweeter on the palate than you may realize.

Some simple substitutions can go a long way here; for example, frozen vegetables are generally much healthier in this regard than canned. And anytime you can swing the "homemade" version of a pasta sauce, a vegetable dip, a canned good, or a lunch meat, it's a very big step in the direction toward limiting the amount of sodium that Toddler, and the rest of your family, will encounter.

Special Toddler Foods

Next in line on the shelf of your grocer's baby food aisle, right by the cereals and jars of first foods, you will find boxes of little mini-meals that resemble old-fashioned TV dinners. These prepackaged toddler meals are supposed to be for the child who has graduated from the softer stuff and is ready for real food. But calling the contents of these products "real food" is a little like calling airplane food a "real meal." Sure, the food items are present, but they are so processed for shipping and storage that the natural flavors are almost completely eroded.

The entrées in the Gerber line include cheese ravioli and tomato sauce with carrots, peas, and corn; chicken and noodles with green beans; macaroni and cheese with peas and carrots; mashed potatoes and gravy with roast chicken; and pasta in meat sauce with green beans. There are also new side dishes "taste-tested by toddlers." (I'd love to meet the toddlers who approved these.) "No Preservatives!" the labels proudly claim, giving another false impression of the healthfulness of these foods. Just check out the sodium content: upwards of 400 milligrams per serving package is common. The products that I tried to eat were so soused with thickeners (cornstarch, tapioca starch) that the meats, noodles, and vegetables were practically identical in terms of taste. The green beans had such a heavily processed taste that they were, to me at least, inedible, making me wonder what impression of fresh vegetables children exposed to these dishes would form.

I have yet to figure out who the market for these products actually is, as they are more expensive (about $2.50 each) than toddler-size portions of homemade meals, and not at all what any parents who want their children to begin to appreciate the true taste of vegetables or fresh meat would have them eat. I'm sure the major promotional message touts convenience, although these dinners still must be heated in the microwave before serving. It doesn't take a whole lot longer to speed-cook a fresh vegetable or warm up leftovers from a previous meal. Sure, the packaging is handy, but you can make and freeze or refrigerate your own prepacked fresh meals by using a couple of pieces of Tupperware. So what's the point?

You'll also find available other toddler items, such as cereal bars, fruit bars, finger food puffs, and even a "juice treats fruit medley" that is billed as "a delicious once-in-a-while treat for toddlers." This actually amounts to little more than toddler candy, with 17 grams of sugar per one-ounce serving, and an ingredients list that includes corn syrup, sugar, and white grape juice concentrate. (Remember what that means in terms of flavor: sweet, sweet, and more sweet.) I have noted earlier that I am not at all opposed to Toddler enjoying bites of occasional desserts and treats as we all do, but, in the interest of training her little palate to recognize a proper level of sweetness, these should be in the form of more adult-palatable foods.

The finger food puffs are more savory and consist almost entirely of rice, corn, or wheat flour, starch, and a little sugar. They carry attractive sounding names such as apple, peach, cherry, strawberry, and apple, but note that all of that "fruit" flavoring is actually produced by peach, cherry, or another kind of powder.

I can't think of any good reason to buy and serve these prepackaged toddler foods, but I can give you one more very good reason to resist, and that has to do with our own parental willpower. For every specialty toddler product that you resist buying today, it will be that much easier to hold the line against the onslaught of kiddie foods that will be coming at you and your child in a very short time. In another year or so, as your child becomes a preschooler with even more of an opinion on what he wants to eat each day, you may reach a point where it will seem as though food marketers have actually moved into your home, designing products tailor-made to his desires. I am constantly amazed at how Willie can see something advertised on television or for sale in a grocery store one time, and immediately relate to it and want it. Walk away now from these kid-friendly boxes that contain packaged, lesser-tasting varieties of foods that you want them to eat. Believe me, it will only get harder, not easier, in the future.

On the Road with Toddler in Tow

"Once in a blue moon, if we're on the road, we might stop at a fast food place. We prefer things like taco trucks in the city if we're traveling."
Chef Gayle Pirie, Foreign Cinema Restaurant, San Francisco, mother of a nine-year-old and a three-year-old

*"We go to fast food restaurants a lot, especially when we're traveling.
I love the idea of trying to stop and find a cute sandwich shop or
something different along the way, but it just takes too much time.
Knowing us, we'd end up getting lost, so we never venture too far
from the major highway."*
Kate, mom to a seven-year-old and a three-year-old

The family vacation, for many, places fast food meals right up there with the license plate game and calls from the backseat of "Mom, he hit me!" as part of the experience. Many families are fine with the idea of eating out at new places when they get to their final destination, but what happens during those days or nights on the road? Enter fast food restaurants, the concept of which takes on a whole new meaning when you don't have travel time to spare.

As part of a family that takes a fair number of long car trips each year, I can completely relate to this situation. I have driven along many an interstate, hopeful (usually to no avail) that the next exit will bring some variety in the food choices available. And, depending on the hunger level and general disposition of my kids, I have more often than not just given up and stopped for a Big Mac or a Whopper. Just about all of the hamburger–French fries–soft drink orders they've ever experienced have been a part of one of these trips.

Fast food outlets scattered along the highways serve the purpose of convenience, which is often the number one priority for people on the road. The kids know what they are getting to eat, which helps to minimize disruptions from tired little ones who may already be off of their schedules. The food is relatively cheap, it's easy to get to, and, most important to harried travelers, the time spent eating amounts to little more than a quick pit stop. Travel by air is the same way; you need to feed the kids en route, so you pick up something from a fast food vendor at the airport.

The predictable consequence of this, of course, is that "fast food chains" and "travel" become synonymous in kids' minds. Is this OK, I've sometimes wondered? Does limiting fast food to certain occasions, such as travel-only, run the risk of turning it all into a "treat"?

There are parents who will tell you that this whole scenario can be avoided by simple planning and better organization than I seem to be able to pull off. Healthful and better-tasting snacks and meals can be prepared at home and brought along on the ride. We often used this strategy on Willie and Daniel during long trips: if we're leaving early in the morning, we pack their cereal and fruit breakfast in a little plastic container and tell them that it's for eating at a certain time—a least 100 miles down the road, or when we are finally seated on the airplane, ready for takeoff. They get milk in a sippy cup when we leave the house to ward off extreme hunger, and then they get to look forward to having breakfast later. I cannot tell you how many minutes of peace and satisfaction this has brought to some otherwise stressful trips.

Beyond that, I've never been good at preplanning kids' meals to eat while on the road or in the air. Instead, I do try—*try*—to make it a point to stop at slightly off-the-beaten-path places when traveling by car. If we do have the luxury of being able to factor the extra time into our travel schedule, we take advantage of it.

One option, particularly good for snacking, is roadside fruit and vegetable stands that are often located near gas stations and rest stops along the highway, especially in the summertime. Fortuitous stops have brought us many a beautiful peach, baskets of cherries and plums, and just-picked apples. Of course you can't count on these places being open or accessible when you need them, but if you do happen to stumble upon them, they are usually a terrific find.

For more complete meals while traveling, you do have to look a bit to find something other than standard fast food, and perhaps incorporate the planning of eating stops into your driving schedule. This works best when you're driving through an area that is well-known for a certain type of cuisine. We've sought out crabs when driving along the Chesapeake Bay, Pennsylvania Dutch fare in the Amish country, fish in Montana, and regional barbecue everywhere from the Carolinas to Wyoming. We've also lucked out on wonderful local mom-and-pop restaurants in small towns along the way. But you do have to take the time to look for them.

And what about when you arrive at your destination? Does the stress of travel and the new, unfamiliar surroundings play havoc with children's good eating? Unfortunately, this is often the case, according to Chef John Brand, the father of three young boys and the executive chef of Las Canarias Restaurant, located in La Mansion del Rio Hotel in San Antonio. He's seen first-hand what many kids eat when they're on vacation, both in his own family and in the families that dine at his hotel restaurant.

"I've noticed that when a lot of parents travel with their kids, they default to the easy, predictable stuff, even when they're in a new place with a lot of interesting regional dishes available," Brand said. "Even here in San Antonio, where we offer great Mexican foods that kids would probably love, people end up asking for the side of fries or a hamburger. I think they just don't want to deal with another hassle when they travel. It's really a shame. The food could be a great learning experience."

Make It Fast

"We went to McDonald's on the way back from Wisconsin the other day, and my son had chicken nuggets. That is a treat. I've got nothing against McDonald's, but if I eat there once every two years, what I notice when I eat is how salty and rich and fatty it is. And it doesn't

*make me feel good. But when I was a kid, I thought McDonald's
was the best thing that ever existed."*
Chef Dan Sachs, Bin 36 and A Mano Trattoria Restaurants,
Chicago, father of three children

For those times when there is nothing else, or you don't have the time or energy to look for anything else, or on those days when, hey, your kids are asking for nothing more than a burger and fries, there will always be a McDonald's. For many families, fast food and chain restaurants like this are a standard and for almost all of us, at least a sometimes-spot. And the food that they serve can certainly have a place in our lives: chain restaurants like this aren't pretending to serve haute cuisine, after all. They know you're there primarily for the convenience, and perhaps the price.

If fast food is what's on tap for your brood for a particular meal, either by request or default, go and guide your kids in making their food selections, encouraging some variety in eating, even here. All of the major fast food chains have made great strides in recent years in adding more healthful and interesting items to their menus. The competition has been good for all of them, forcing chain restaurants to differentiate themselves from one another with new products, cooking methods, and flavorings. Consumer response, for the most part, has been very good, as sales at all of the major national chains are up and are predicted to continue rising for the next few years.[47]

If your family stops at fast food places often, then this should be a time to think "healthful" and "varied" as much as possible, rather than completely letting your children's taste buds lead them. As in any other restaurant, don't automatically start with the kiddie menus. Remember the Big Three palate dimmers, and how they abound at these places: fries and many of the sandwiches are loaded with fat and sodium; soft drinks and added condiments such as ketchup contain the sweet sugar taste. If you're trying to steer clear of these, look for something fresh, such as salads. Also, the chicken products are usually "better" than beef hamburgers, both in nutritional value and in flavor profile. The chicken sandwiches and salad selections will have more of a true meat flavor than will hamburgers, particularly if they are grilled, because of the chicken's lower natural fat content, as compared to the level in beef. Hamburgers made of beef, with its marbling and higher fat content, tend to taste more like . . . fat.

So if your kids always ask for the same type of hamburger, have them try a chicken sandwich. If they always eat a certain type of chicken sandwich, order it grilled, or in a salad. Try skipping the fries in favor of a small salad, carrot sticks, apple slices, or a fruit cup, or, failing that, place a smaller order for fries and let them all share. Pass on the sodas and order water or milk to drink. Think variety, and you will do a little better in these places. Any time that you can offer your kids something new to eat, it will be beneficial to them, even if it's in the same basic package.

What about Juice?

"My daughter is the only child I know who doesn't get juice at home. Friends have said, 'Oh, that's so great that your daughter doesn't drink juice; how do you do it?' Well, I just don't buy the stuff. What you do and don't have in the house is the first line of defense."
Jennifer, mom to a three-year-old

"The big thing that makes me crazy about children's birthday parties is that everyone seems to serve juice. Parties are now synonymous in my kids' minds with juice boxes."
Marilyn, mother of three-and-a-half-year-old twin boys

For some reason that completely escapes me, many toddlers seem to live on juice as their beverage of choice. In fact, by the time they reach their first birthday, almost 90% of American children have had juice.[48] On a daily basis, half of all kids ages two to five take in 148 calories each day by drinking 11.1 ounces of juice.[49] Those numbers are up, incidentally, from 1994 numbers, when kids received a daily dose of 135 calories from 9.9 ounces of juice.

Orange juice, apple juice, grape juice, fruit punches of some sort; check out the sippy cup, and most likely, that's what you'll find. Maybe, because of years of marketing and parental conditioning, so many people believe that these are not only the best drinks to serve young children, but the only beverages that kids can or will consume.

If you read the small print, you'll learn that there really is a difference between "fruit juices" and "fruit drinks" or other terms that are used. In order to be labeled as a juice, a product must be 100% fruit juice, and if reconstituted from concentrate, the label must state so. Any beverages that are less than 100% fruit juice are called a fruit "drink" or fruit "beverage" or even fruit "cocktail." These "drinks" can be anywhere from 10% to 99% real juice; the balance is made up of added sweeteners and other flavorings or vitamin fortifiers. All ingredients are listed on the label.

The handy packaging, the palatable taste, the variety of colors and flavors available, the pretty pictures of whole fruit on the labels—yes, you'd think that juice is the perfect beverage for toddlers and young children. But is it?

Pediatricians give a tepid OK. A 2001 policy statement by the American Academy of Pediatrics (AAP) states up front that "although juice consumption has some benefits, it also has potential detrimental effects," including the contribution to tooth decay, diarrhea, and even malnutrition. (Even the title of this paper, *The Use and Misuse of Fruit Juice in Pediatrics,* tells you something.) These doctors go on to state that fruit juice should only be served to kids as part of a meal or snack, and that four to six ounces per day is "more than adequate."

"Fruit juices and fruit drinks are easily over-consumed by toddlers and young children because they taste good," the AAP paper concludes. And by "good," in this instance, you better believe they mean "sweet."

There is mounting evidence that juice—particularly children's juices—may not be nutritionally beneficial at all. Remove the fiber that you get by eating the fruit whole, and you're left with a liquid that has a very high sugar content. Yes, there are vitamins as well, but these can, and should, be obtained in food form. The consumption of just six ounces a day of 100% fruit juice was associated with weight gain and a lack of growth in 94 two-year-olds who participated in a 1997 study in New York.[50] And a lot of kids are drinking a whole lot more than that.

I gathered my foodie/chef group together for a juice tasting, similar to the baby food session we conducted for the previous chapter. (I'm sure these people are ready to write me off forever as a hostess.) Using our best stemware and evaluation techniques, we rated the taste, packaging, and color of many of the commercial juices marketed specifically for kids. No fancy wine tasting was ever more thorough. We realized that, while we all have kids and many of us drink adult juices ourselves, it had been a long time since we'd tasted the kiddie versions, if we'd ever done so at all. So we sampled from about twenty different jars, including grape juice, apple juice, carrot juice, berry juices, combination juices, and more.

The first thing we noted about most of these products, particularly the ones geared at infants and toddlers, is their "off" aroma (to use a wine term). Give them a good whiff, and you'll find that the odor (the "nose," for you oenophiles) bears some resemblance to what you would expect it to be—but somehow it's just not quite right. Most of these juices are really pungent—a little like fruit gone bad, past its prime, or what is found in an imitation version, rather than a nice fresh piece.

Also, we were knocked over by the sweetness in all of these kids' juices. If you think adult orange, apple, or cranberry juice is sweet, just try a sip of a children's product. And no wonder: a close look at the labels—in small type, opposite the cartoons and colorful lettering—reveals the high quantity of sugar. The information is presented in grams, with the hope, I suppose, that most American parents have no idea what this means in terms of volume.

Most of the juice labels that you see make mention of the fact that the product contains "no added sugar" or is "100% natural juice." Oh, great, you may think; this must mean that this juice is the most healthful. But take a closer look. The sugar content, measured in grams, will inevitably be very high. And if the sugar content is high, you can bet that the beverage is super-sweet on the palate. How can that be, if they aren't adding any? Remember that there are different kinds of sugar. Sucrose is the white stuff that you usually think of when you hear the word "sugar." Fructose is the natural sugar contained in fruits such as apples, bananas, and berries. Added or natural, it's all sugar to your body, and to your palate. It makes the beverage taste really sweet.

Most kid's juices contain a *lot* of sugar—anywhere from 25 to 34 grams per cup, or even more. To translate that into something familiar, 34 grams of sugar is the equivalent of 8.5 teaspoons of sugar. So as you're pouring that small bit of juice (and remember, a serving is just eight ounces, or one cup) into a plastic cup or bottle, just visualize yourself dumping eight-plus teaspoons of sugar in with that liquid. (I know. Ew.)

Juices that are marketed more as "adult beverages," like grapefruit, berry, or some orange juices, are high in sugar, too; don't get me wrong. But the corresponding whole fruits are more tart in flavor, naturally, than are bananas, apples, and grapes, making the flavors of those juices more in balance, and more identical to that of the whole fruit.

Here is what we found in our taste test of some of the leading juices.

WHITE GRAPE JUICE

There it is, with that cute and familiar Gerber baby on the label, a white grape juice for . . . babies? No, although you'd never know it by reading the label, where no mention is made of the fact that AAP emphatically states that juices should not be given to babies less than six months of age. A call to the consumer product hotline confirms that no mention of this fact is made on the product; however, the Gerber Web site does clarify the age recommendation. "And parents should always ask their pediatricians before giving Baby each new food, including juice," the hotline attendant told me. (Of course we should, but how many of us do?)

This beverage had a bland, watery aroma and very little grape flavor, yet just four ounces (one-half of a cup) contains 180 calories and 20 grams of sugar.

A comparable white grape juice by Nestle, Juicy Juice, is more clearly aimed at older children. This label touts a partnership with *Scholastic* magazines—convenient if you're looking for an entrée to present product materials to schools and teachers, right? There was actually a little difference between the flavor of this juice and that of the Gerber version. It's slightly "grapier" in aroma and has a tangier taste. And there is a little less sugar; an eight-ounce serving (one cup) contains 150 calories and 34 grams of sugar.

While I'm on the subject of white grape juice, it's interesting to note that a version of this product is actually used by food manufacturers as a sweetener for other foods! Concentrated grapes and the liquid juice that they produce are very, very sweet;

so sweet that they can be used in commercial products such as jams and baked goods as a "natural sugar." That, alone, is reason to never give a young child this beverage.

APPLE JUICE

In another kid-oriented product "tie-in," Apple & Eve presents Big Bird's Apple Juice, complete with a picture and "fun facts" about this Sesame Street character. The juice itself has some semblance of an apple aroma but is very weak on flavor and has little actual apple taste. Eight ounces (one cup) provides 110 calories and 22 grams of sugar.

Gerber has an Apple Juice, too, that is very sweet, with an off-aroma and no apple flavor that we could discern. Four ounces (one-half cup) of this product—obviously aimed at the youngest of children—provides 60 calories and 13 grams of sugar. We also tried an apple juice by Earth's Best, which adds a "#2" symbol to the juice jar label to identify this product as suitable for babies over the age of six months. With "just" 11 grams of sugar in four ounces, and 55 calories, this juice is organic (and therefore, pro-moted as a more healthful product). As far as the actual flavor of the product, however, there is neither an apple aroma nor a distin-guishable apple taste.

Finally, we also tried a Lite Apple Juice, sweetened with Splenda (sucralose), a sugar substitute that is chemically derived from sugar. Interestingly, this was determined to be the most true-apple-flavored of all of apple juices sampled, and it had less of the sweet aroma that is so prevalent in the others. But it did have a very strong chemical-tasting finish, thanks to the Splenda. This juice has 25 calories per eight ounce cup and six grams of sugar.

APPLE-BANANA JUICE

The addition of banana adds even more sweetness to the flavor of all of these juices. Gerber's Apple-Banana Juice has an extremely sweet aroma and taste, as well as an unpleasant lingering after-taste. It touts 14 grams of sugar in just four ounces. The Nestle Apple-Banana Juicy Juice has more of a tart, apple odor, but also has a very sweet flavor and aftertaste, with 120 calories and 27 grams of sugar in one cup here.

APPLE-CARROT JUICE

We tried First Juice's Apple and Carrot juice, which actually contains pear and pineapple in addition to the named fruits. The label reads "50% less sugar"; that translates into 12 grams and 50 calories in the eight-ounce cup. This juice is very bright in color (orange), leading us to believe that the flavor would be similarly intense. Surprise here; it was actually one of the most bland. It tasted mostly like water, with a weak pear-like addition.

Our testing group was surprised by these results, as we had assumed that these children's juices would be more like juices that adults more typically drink in their flavor accuracy. But we were disappointed to find that virtually all of the kids' juices that we tested smell and taste nothing like the fruit that they are supposed to contain. When I drink a glass of grapefruit or orange or carrot juice, the flavor that I get is fairly similar to the flavor of the whole fruit or vegetable. That's simply not the case with these kids' products.

We can all feel good about giving our kids fruit, but don't believe for a minute that these commercial juices are in any way a substitute, either in terms of nutritional value or in teaching them to appreciate what real fruits taste like. "Children should be encouraged to eat whole fruits to meet their recommended daily fruit intake," AAP says. Amen to that.

If you want your kids to love the taste of fruit down the road, spare yourself the expense, and your kids these flavor abominations, and give them their apples, grapes, bananas, and such in the "real" form. Another common parental practice is to dilute juices with water, lightening up the beverage and reducing the amount of sugar and calories consumed per fluid ounce. I encourage you also to avoid this practice; you're still just reinforcing the message to Toddler that beverages must be flavored in some way to taste good.

Why am I making such a big deal about this?

Because once a child, or an adult for that matter, becomes accustomed to sweet beverages, it is hard to accept them in any other fashion. Think about how this may be true even for yourself: do you like your coffee prepared in a certain manner? If you like to add cream, sugar, or an artificial sweetener, it's probably the first thing you reach for when you get a new cup, before even taking a sip of the beverage. My friend Susan says that she is "addicted to sweet tea," and won't drink it any other way. How about people who always drink the same soda, be it diet or regular, simply because they are used to it and like a standard taste? See how difficult it can be to retrain the palate once it comes to expect a food or beverage to taste a certain way?

And just consider how much juice the average toddler drinks in a day: 3.8 ounces, or almost half a cup, for two-year-olds, and 4.6 ounces, well over half a cup, for most three-year-olds.[51] That may not seem like so much in comparison with the amount of beverages an adult normally consumes, but remember that these are children and this is *every day*. Is it any wonder that American children grow up to be American teens who find sweet sodas so appealing?

I cannot emphasize this enough: with their inherent sweetness, juices for children this age are, for the most part, a "gateway beverage" to soda, which, as we have seen in the Feeding Infants and Toddlers Survey results and other studies, is consumed far too often by too many children and teens. If you take nothing else away from this chapter, I encourage you to severely restrict the amount of juice that your toddler consumes, and if possible, eliminate it completely from his diet. The sugar content in juice is just too high for toddlers to consume on a regular basis. A steady diet of juice will, more quickly than just about anything else, "numb the palate" and teach your child that all beverages should be sweet. What should he be drinking instead? Milk (skim or reduced fat, according to your doctor's instructions), or water. Lots and lots of water.

In my many interviews with America's top chefs about what they are feeding their own kids, the one thing that most of them consistently put on the "never consume" list is juice. I found it interesting that so many chefs, who presumably have an even more vested interest than the rest of us in getting their kids to eat and enjoy a wide range of foods, make juice off-limits for their young children. Chicago restaurateur Dan Sachs, a former chef in New York and London and the father of three, adamantly stated: "We never have juice really, only maybe occasionally fresh-squeezed juice. That's one thing I do put my foot down on. We're all about water, water, and more water."

Adds Marc Murphy of New York's Landmarc Restaurant, "My kids (five years and 21 months) don't know what soda is. To them, it's like beer; it's for adults. My daughter does like sparkling water and, when she's in the restaurant, something that she calls Princess Juice, which is a splash of cranberry juice in club soda. But other than that, it's all milk and water." Hugh Matheson, chef and owner of The Kitchen in Boulder, Colorado, said of his five-year-old twin sons: "They're not allowed juice; just water. My criteria is to avoid added sugar, juices, and caffeine." And this from Barbara Black, owner of Black Salt in Washington, D.C.: "We make lemonade every once in a while, but mostly they [her two young sons] drink a lot of water and milk, that sort of thing. We don't juice anything."

If all of this seems too draconian for your house, just remember this: at around the age of two or three, when your youngster really starts to socialize with other kids—hits the birthday party circuit, or starts in regular playgroups or nursery school, for example—he or she will be presented with servings of juice at every turn. I can promise you that other parents, teachers, coaches, and caregivers will give out boxes of juice with abandon. A no-exceptions "we don't buy juice or have it at home" rule will limit your child's consumption considerably, without totally alienating him from what the other kids are doing.

And finally, for good measure, if you really must serve juice, a few summarizing cautions from AAP:

1. *Never* give juice to babies before the age of six months;

2. Don't serve juice from bottles or sippy cups, or anything else that makes it easy to tote around;

3. Limit juice intake for toddlers and young children to four to six ounces per day, at the most. (Remember, this is less than one cup.)

4. Remember that fruit *drinks* are even worse than fruit *juice*. Read those labels!

What I've Learned

— As Baby turns into Toddler, he can give you a real shock by also morphing into a Picky Eater. A lot of psychological head games concerning food acceptance can start during the toddler years. Obviously, it's best to work with your toddler to get her through this stage, rather than battle with her, as much as you possibly can.

— Eat with your kids, as much and as often as you possibly can, even at this stage. Set schedules that work best for your family.

— By the time they turn one, or shortly thereafter, children should be eating essentially what you eat. (This is presuming your diet to be generally nutritious and healthful, and rich in variety and flavor!)

— The early eating years are actually the best time to encourage your child to eat a lot of new foods. Take advantage of this and, should food ruts and picky eater behavior start during the toddler years, continue to offer a variety of foods with the confidence that this, too, shall pass.

— "Kid-friendly" restaurants, menus, and the like are not the answer! In fact, they are at the root of the problem.

— Ditto for children's breakfast cereals consumed on a regular basis, and just about any other food product designed and marketed especially for kids.

— You can find something for your kids to eat other than hamburgers, French fries, and sodas at fast food restaurants.

— Skip the juice!

CHAPTER 6

⌘

The Preschooler: A Real Little Eater

By the time your child reaches the age of three or four, he can probably tell you and anyone else who will listen exactly what he does and doesn't like to eat. But ask him again in a month or two, and you may get a different answer.

At this stage in the game, picky eater traits that first manifested themselves in the infant and toddler years may intensify or let up, kids with an interest in cooking may want to spend more time helping out in the kitchen, and those who have worn the Good Eater label all of their lives may suddenly turn on you. These are the years that parents realize how quickly likes, dislikes, and habits can change, as their kids grow up a bit and begin to absorb more influences from the outside world. And the parent who is used to complete command over what his child eats may be in for a rude awakening at this point, as our kids' food choices seem to be one of the first things we lose control over.

With little experience in how to pick the best foods for a proper diet, however, kids at this age are hardly in a position to be calling the shots. So hang in there in the effort to provide high-quality, flavorful meals! It can be quite discouraging when you realize that you no longer have complete say-so over what your child eats, nor are you the only voice on the topic that he will hear. But stick with it, and if nothing else, fall back on the "but that's what we do at home" rule. Believe me, your kids will learn enough about all the food options that exist without you bringing questionable or objectionable products into your home, or taking them to eat at places you normally wouldn't eat yourself.

"But What Does It Taste Like?"

"I think it helps to get kids thinking about what they are eating. My son can tell when a vinaigrette is off-balance; he knows when it has too much vinegar in it. That comes from me talking to him about it: 'Tell me what you taste. Is it salty? Is it sweet? Do you think it has too much olive oil?'"
Chef Robbie Lewis, Bacar Restaurant, San Francisco, father of a five-year-old and a two-and-a-half-year-old

Parents, we can most likely agree, have the responsibility to train and educate their children on how to make smart decisions in life. With this in mind as it applies to diet, nutrition, and the enjoyment of eating, now is the perfect time to start really talking to your kids about their food. Where does it all come from? How is it grown or raised? How does it make its way onto our plates? If you think you don't know enough about this yourself, not to fear: as long as you have the interest, the information is increasingly available as more and more Americans want to learn about the origins of their food. A simple trip to the produce aisle of the grocery store or to a farmer's market can be an interesting experience for a young child, if you take the time to talk about what is around you.

Get in the habit of asking your preschooler about the food that she eats, using open-ended questions that require a bit of contemplation and reasoning, rather than the more common "Do you like that?" or "Is it good?" (Too much potential for the conversation to die with the word "No!") Ask kids to describe the flavors of what they are eating, even if it's something that they've had a hundred times in the past. After taking a bite and chewing, have them pause before swallowing and consider: Is it salty? Sweet? Sharp, or bitter? Do you taste the orange juice in that sauce, the capers in the egg salad, the olives on the pizza? Can you taste that pickle I added to your sandwich? What is that smell coming from the oven? Ask kids to compare the taste of green grapes and red grapes, or if they can tell the difference between the cantaloupe and the honeydew and the watermelon in their fruit salad. Their reflections and answers are not as important as the fact that they are stopping to consider the question, and the flavors of their foods.

Talk about the texture of different foods, the way they smell and feel, on the hands and to the tongue. Some foods are sticky, some are slippery, others are crunchy or creamy. Sometimes it's the food itself that has these characteristics, and sometimes it's in the way that it's been cooked. And here's a big one: the heat level of different foods. Teach Preschooler the difference between food that is *spicy* hot and food that is *temperature* hot. If it's just come from the oven, for example, you may need to wait a minute for it to cool off enough to enjoy. But a spicy dish, such as a salsa or a hot pepper or hot sausage, will remain warm to the tongue even if served at room temperature.

These are all beginner steps in what culinary types refer to as the education of the palate, guiding a taster toward flavor that is superior and away from those that are inferior, and learning to discern between the two. It's not at all hard to put into practice in your own life; just look at ordinary day-to-day eating experiences as opportunities for your kids to pay attention to what they are *tasting*, rather than just what they are *eating*. If you stop by a bakery or make homemade cookies, talk about why these taste so much better than a packaged variety. ("Do you taste the creamy butter? Doesn't the chocolate taste fresh?") Talk about foods blending together and complementing each other. ("Do you like that spicy mustard on your hot dog? Can you taste the smoky flavor from the grill?" "You like avocadoes and tomatoes; try this guacamole!") Foods that fail the test should be mentioned, too, as in: "This candy must be really old; can you tell how it tastes stale?" "Oh, these French fries are really greasy; you taste oil more than potato! Do you feel how the oil coats your tongue?" "This cereal has a lot less sugar than that cereal; you can really tell what grains taste like!" And so on.

An important part of coaxing along a child's palate is to make foods and certain dishes special by emphasizing their seasonality and freshness. Ideally, they should only be served at appropriate times of the year. Strawberries, spinach, and asparagus always taste best in the spring; peaches, tomatoes, and zucchini in summertime; apple pies and squashes in the fall; warming, comfort food recipes and root vegetables during the cold winter months.

"We go to the farmer's market and we'll talk about seasonality," said Chef Lewis of San Francisco, who cooks at the modern American restaurant and wine bar Bacar. His son Dante, age five, will ask, "Why can't we have strawberries?" "And I'll say, 'Because they're not in season right now,'" Lewis says. "And we'll talk about: what are seasons? Things are tasty during this time of year because they're happiest when it's warm, and they're not happy in the winter, so they don't grow well and they're not so tasty. We're engaged about why food is and when it is."

It goes without saying that all of this can best be accomplished by buying only "fresh" produce, but if that's not possible, at least try to follow this example and set seasonal relationships and expectations around food. Does Grandmother have a special Thanksgiving side dish? "We only get this during the holidays!" Does a backyard cookout with hamburgers on the grill and watermelon slices sound like the perfect Fourth of July menu? Create traditions by serving this menu every year as your family's holiday celebration. Seasonality and superior flavor go hand in hand.

Imparting Flavor

"I'm hoping that this is just a quirky phase, but my daughter has become a habitual condiment eater. She wants ketchup on everything."
Post on parenting Web site

Try to make this a rule when you're preparing or choosing foods for your kids: pay attention to flavor as much as possible, whenever possible, in every way possible. No matter what you're serving, even if it's something simple like a sandwich or some pasta, or even a prepackaged dinner, do what you can to improve the true flavor of the food. This is not as hard as it sounds, and it's something that you can get good at very quickly by adding your own enhancements.

Chefs refer to this technique as "layering flavors." What this means is that good cooks know how to select particular foods and herbs and spices to be served together in a recipe, because of the way that they complement and enhance each other. It means that the total flavor of a dish is greater than the sum of the individual parts. Cherries, for example, are wonderful, all by themselves. So is lamb. But combine the two by preparing a sauce for the lamb that is made of cherries, olive oil, shallots, and chopped sage, and you have a real winner. Then serve this lamb with cherry sauce over rice made with chicken stock and with diced preserved lemon, and you have a dish to remember.

Think of it like an artist painting a picture, or a composer writing a symphony. One color or a few lone notes are pretty bland; start adding complementing elements, however, and soon you have a masterpiece. It's all in the skill of the craftsman as to how well the painting or musical score comes together. It's very possible, of course, to go overboard with this and end up with a real mess on your hands. And it's the same thing with cooking, so start working on your flavor savvy when your kids are with you. Practice is the best teacher.

Remember that proper flavor building refers to the introduction of new, well-paired elements to a recipe. Not to be confused with this is the "blind" addition of condiments to foods. Flavor building does not involve simply adding something that you know your child will like (especially one of the Big Three) to make a dish acceptable to him! Ketchup, mayonnaise, salad dressing, chocolate syrups, dipping sauce, barbecue or steak sauce—there is no end to the bottled, processed products that you can buy to doctor up food. Appropriately used, of course, added condiments complement foods and appeal to kids, but watch out! It is easy to overuse them, especially if you've reached a point of conflict with the meal. Allow too heavy a pour, and on too many items, and before long, it's the condiment that's becoming the focus of the flavor, rather than the item on which it was slopped.

Condiments can be a real bane to a child's flavor development, and their proliferated use usually starts about this age. So no matter what you're serving, try, as much as possible, to cut down on the use of added condiments. The most obvious example and biggest offender in American children's diets is ketchup, which seems to "flavor" everything kids eat, from hot dogs to French fries to scrambled eggs and even macaroni and cheese. What's so bad about it? Well, besides the fact that condiments add unnecessary sugars and calories, they also have "false flavors" that mask, rather than enhance, the taste of the food. You may have seen kids who insist on adding ketchup or some such condiment to every dish they eat, and refuse to eat certain foods without it. Don't fall into the trap of making it OK for everything to taste like ketchup, or any other condiment.

When you allow ketchup to be dumped onto every food, less-than-desirable foods to be slathered with butter or cheese, or bacon bits to be sprinkled everywhere, you are allowing sugar or fat or sodium to be a *cover* for the base food. Vegetables are a prime example of this. Kids need to learn to appreciate the taste of individual vegetables, even the very bitter ones, so flavor layering should *enhance*, rather than *mask*, the natural taste. Steaming or microwaving raw vegetables such as carrots, green beans, or cauliflower in a little bit of chicken stock, rather than water, will draw out the natural flavors of the vegetables. Pouring melted cheese over baked potatoes or broccoli, or covering a tossed salad with fatty dressing, on the other hand, simply disguises the natural flavor of the vegetables.

Give the flavor-building concept a try, and have some fun with it. When you eat out at a restaurant, pay attention to the way the chef put the dishes together. You can learn a lot from these pros. Fortunately, the vast majority of kids at this age, probably yours included, are hardly connoisseurs of fine food and cooking, and they will cut you a lot of slack if you fail. And remember that the goal of this is not to force yourself to learn to cook if you don't want to, but just to expose your children to as wide a variety of flavors as possible.

Here are some ideas that work well with foods that kids this age usually like.

♦ Cook rice, couscous, or pasta in low-sodium chicken, beef, or vegetable stock rather than water. Orange juice also works well, although because of the thickness of the liquid, you'll need to make that about half juice and half water. Finish with chopped fresh herbs, such as parsley or basil, and a little bit of salt and pepper.

♦ If you're making sandwiches, skip the store-bought mayonnaise and regular yellow mustard and substitute a more flavorful spread, such as Dijon mustard, or horseradish-flavored mayonnaise.

♦ What about hamburgers and hot dogs? If you're whipping up the hamburger meat at home, you can go all out with the additions to the ground meat, as the list of herbs and spices that work well in hamburgers is practically endless. Curry powder, allspice, Chinese five-spice powder, ginger, cumin, turmeric, nutmeg; just go through your spice rack and think about what works well together. Don't get too crazy though; this is an example of how a good idea can go south in a hurry if too many conflicting flavors are added. Hot dogs are a kids' staple that can be jazzed up by grilling or broiling rather than boiling, and paying attention to the type of relish or mustard that you use as topping.

♦ Use chopped fresh herbs as a way to add flavor to pre-prepared, store-bought foods. A jar of spaghetti sauce, for instance, or even canned SpaghettiOs, will taste better if sprinkled liberally with chopped parsley or oregano. Add a surprise to ice cream: a chopped light herb, like tarragon, lavender, or mint, is delicious and much more interesting that just coating it with chocolate syrup. Chopped fresh herbs also work well in yogurt.

♦ Don't be afraid to add sharp-tasting flavor enhancers like garlic or onions to foods. If you need to tone down the amount added for the kids, that's fine, but they should become familiar with the taste of these staples.

♦ Shake things up a little by serving new flavors in unexpected places. If your kids are used to cinnamon toast for breakfast, for example, try substituting ground ginger for the cinnamon. If it's always peanut butter and jelly sandwiches, a new nut spread, like cashew butter or almond butter, may be an interesting change.

♦ If you're serving them frozen things like fish sticks or chicken nuggets, try for a topping or dip more interesting than the usual ketchup. How about fresh salsa or guacamole?

♦ If it's Friday night, it must be pizza night, and even this staple-in-most-household-menus can get a fresh, flavorful twist. Try one with a whole-wheat crust, or topped with basil pesto sauce rather than tomato sauce. Toppings should vary from week to week, too—a lot.

♦ Experiment with more adult-oriented condiments such as vinegars, fish, or oyster sauce, toasted nuts, and different oils like safflower or toasted sesame. Keep on hand Asian bottled sauces, such as hoisin and garlic-ginger sauce, and Latin favorites, such as chipotle peppers in adobo sauce. Bottled hot sauces, used in moderation, can add interest. Most kids will like the flavors that any of these add to recipes, as long as they are introduced slowly and in quantities less than what adults may use. Balsamic vinegar, especially, is a real hit at my house.

♦ You can do wonders with fresh lemon and lime juice. Keep these on hand, and use them when cooking or reheating meats or grains, such as rice and couscous.

I'm also a big fan of using lemon or lime peel in cooking; it adds an even more concentrated flavor.

♦ The Italians call it gremolata; in Northern Africa, it's known as chermoula, and it's a wonderful flavor blend to have on hand to add to anything from pasta to meat to vegetable dishes. Just combine finely-diced garlic with chopped lemon peel or orange peel, chile flakes if you like a little heat, and fresh parsley. Store in the refrigerator.

♦ Instead of sugar or sweet toppings on cut-up fresh fruits, try balsamic vinegar.

♦ Don't neglect texture when it comes to adding flavors. Stir granola or mixed nuts into ice cream for some added crunch; add some cooling yogurt or sour cream to a hot dish; add crispiness to a soup with dried noodles.

♦ Garnishes are an easy way to add flavor and improve the look of the dish at the same time. Try adding chopped herbs such as parsley to pastas, or cilantro to stir-fries and Mexican recipes. If you live in a small space and have no room for a garden, grow a few favorite herbs in flower pots on the kitchen windowsill.

♦ I love to use beer and wine in sauces that I make, and I don't hesitate to serve those same sauces in dishes that I give to my children. The splash of alcohol that I use adds flavors that can't be duplicated by anything else. This is *not* the same thing as giving children alcohol to drink.

If you're trying to figure out which flavors work well together, think about classic flavor pairings, such as sweet and sour or rich and creamy. Why do people serve fruit and cheese together?

Because of the way the sweet of the fruit and the salty cheese combine. Chocolate and strawberries or coffee and cake are also good examples, as these combine sharp and sweet. Try tasting food or ingredient components individually, to get a taste of the flavor of each part. Bite into a piece of oregano, basil, thyme, or other herb. Put a dab of a couple of different ground spices on the tip of your tongue, and really pay attention to what you sense: Hot? Earthy? Sweet? Nutty? Think about how these can be used to enhance the dish that you are serving.

Are you getting the point? Rather than just serve food in the same, usually bland, way all the time, you can do a lot to step up the flavor experience, even if it's a prepackaged, shortcut meal night.

And finally, a word about the best-known and probably most incorrectly used and most misunderstood seasonings of all: plain old salt and pepper. In the numerous cooking classes that I've taken, the chef instructors have many times made the point that the one thing that the average home cook could do to most improve the taste of his or her meals is to judiciously add salt and pepper, throughout the cooking process. Salt, especially, works to draw out flavors.

I know many home cooks who are afraid to use it because we all know that too much salt in the diet is unhealthful. Likewise, I know people who don't put a bite of food in their mouth before salting the dish, without first tasting it to see if salt is really needed. (On the same note, I find it annoying when restaurant waiters set down a plate of food and immediately ask if I'd like ground pepper on top. How do I know before I've tasted it, and besides, shouldn't I be able to trust the chef to properly season the dish?)

As I've stated many times in this book, too much sodium in the diet is a huge hazard, from a taste as well as a health point of view. But, again, remember this: 80% of the sodium in our diets (children's diets included) comes from processed, canned, and fast foods, *not from properly seasoned dishes prepared with fresh foods.*[52]

Heed the sodium content on any and all of these processed and fast foods that you buy, but don't be afraid to use a little salt in the dishes that you are preparing at home with fresh, raw ingredients. It makes all the difference in enhancing the natural flavor of the foods that you serve.

Someone's in the Kitchen

"My son likes to cook with me, and we do that a lot together. When we are at the market or cooking, I'm very frank about the ingredients. He knows the ham bone in the beans comes from a dead pig. I don't try to put a pretty face on it, nor do I paint butchering as something sad. It is what it is, and that is pretty miraculous."
Niccole, mom to a five-year-old

Given the right introduction to the activity and the freedom to be themselves (read: make a mess), most kids this age love to help out in the kitchen. Kids may have their own toy kitchens, grocery shopping carts, plastic food items, and checkout scanners. They love to lick spoons, stir batter, watch things rise in the oven, and, of course, sample what comes out in the end. And even if you don't like to cook yourself and spend as little time in the kitchen as you possibly can, it never hurts to encourage the activity a bit with your preschooler. You never know; you just might be launching the next Julia Child or Emeril Lagasse. (And then you'd never have to cook again!) Yes, you have to prepare for the chaotic mess that may ensue (one friend refers to cooking sessions with her preschooler and twin toddlers as "Hell's Kitchen"), but when all is baked and eaten, this is probably the single best way to get your kids more interested in their food.

Start by letting your children go to the grocery store or farmer's market with you, at least some of the time. I'm not kidding myself here: there are many times when I am simply in too much of a hurry to add little hands to the shopping process, so I make a point of going to the store when my children are in school or with Dad. But every now and then it's fun for them and can be a good experience, even beyond riding in the car-shaped grocery cart. Tell them that they can pick out one new vegetable to try, or any fruit that is red. Show them how meats look in the package; can you believe this will be the chicken on your plate tonight? Roam the aisles and point out various ingredients that come together to make cookies, lasagna, or a favorite soup.

When you're ready to cook, have your kids pull up little stools or sit at the kitchen table if your counters are too high for them to reach comfortably. Outfit them in pint-size aprons and let them participate as much as possible in the preparation of their food. I do believe that you will see a correlation between their involvement in the cooking, and their willingness to try new foods. If you subscribe to any food magazines or like to look at cookbooks, let your kids thumb through these with you. Willie loves to do this, and he often makes remarks on what "looks good" and which recipes he "wants to try." And let your children help you unpack groceries and put them away. This will teach them about proper food storage techniques, as well as familiarize them with the contents of the refrigerator, freezer, and pantry.

When it comes to cooking and food preparation, assembly foods such as sandwiches and salads are an easy first step; lay out the individual components and let kids put together their own versions. Stirring cake batters, cookie dough, and the like is usually a big hit, too. Let kids help with the washing and drying of fresh fruits and vegetables and the picking of herbs if you have a little garden. It may take a bit of patience on your part to get used to having little hands helping out in the kitchen, and there may be some things that you have to overlook in the name of advancing this budding culinary interest. Willie went through a phase where he insisted on putting his hands all over raw foods such as meats and cookie dough, and I had to bite back from too many rounds of "don't touch!"

Show your kids the different pieces of kitchen equipment that you own and explain what things are used for, even things that seem obvious to you such as whisks, pizza cutters, ice cream scoops, or vegetable peelers. These can be very interesting to young children who have never seen them in operation. Most kids are also fascinated by electrical appliances, especially devices such as food processors, mixers, and blenders, which make a lot of noise. Washington, D.C.-area pastry chef David Guas loves to make fancy desserts with his two sons and says, "I get the most cheering from them if something ignites."

By the way, cooking with their kids is one trick that almost all of the chefs whom I interviewed for this book mentioned as a way to enhance their children's interest in foods. Marc Murphy's (Landmarc Restaurant, New York) five-year-old daughter helps him pick the herbs off of their stems, and cracks eggs for omelets. Colombian native pastry chef Dunia Borga of Alo and La Duni restaurants in Dallas is another chef who loves to cook breakfast with her son. "I love making breakfast and I always bake something fresh on my day off," she says. "Brandon is in charge of making smoothies and fruit salad."

Homemade pizza is always a big hit, says Hugo Matheson of Boulder, Colorado's, The Kitchen restaurant; he often makes it with his young twin sons. Chef Frank Bonnano of Luca d'Italia and Osteria Marca in Denver taught his boys, ages six and four, to roll pasta. "We'll make these really crazy-shaped raviolis and we'll make the ricotta cheese the day before. Then we stuff the pasta with the cheese we've made. We just put butter or olive oil on them, and parmesan cheese, and they love it."

Family cooking has a special meaning for Fred Neuville, chef/owner of the Fat Hen on John's Island, South Carolina, who with his wife has adopted five foster children, ages ten, twelve, thirteen, fifteen, and sixteen. In eight years, he's watched them grow from "never having experienced a fresh vegetable" to "eating just about everything" as they learned to cook with him. "Starting in first grade, they each had to help us make dinner," Neuville said. "Now they all help with washing, peeling, and chopping at home, and the older ones can help with light prep at the restaurant. It's an education they'll carry for the rest of their lives."

I will never forget the drama of last Christmas Eve, when Willie and I were in the kitchen cooking together, making gingerbread cookies to leave for Santa Claus. I was using an old stand mixer that was on its last legs, and as soon as I turned it on, it started crackling and smoking. I probably got a little overexcited as I rushed to unplug the mixer, tiny sparks flying all over the counter. "We might have to call in the firefighters to put this out," I distinctly remember saying. That offhand remark turned out to be most unfortunate, as I had momentarily forgotten that Willie had asked for nothing for Christmas except a fireman's suit. That night before going to bed, he wanted to amend his letter to Santa saying that "he didn't want to be a fireman after all, and to please bring a football player uniform instead." Santa didn't get the message in time.

Fortunately, at least to date, our other kitchen disasters have been confined to recipes that haven't turned out so well, but kitchen safety is definitely an issue. The two greatest risks for young kids are sharp knives and hot ovens. The chefs whom I have talked with, who have probably witnessed some serious kitchen accidents, had a lot to say about this issue when it comes to cooking with their kids.

"My son (Dante, age five) cooks a lot. We're right there so he doesn't burn himself and we teach him what not to touch, or how to touch it, and don't act this way around the kitchen counter, or whatever," says Robbie Lewis of San Francisco's Bacar restaurant. "We have special 'Dante Knives' that aren't as sharp, kind of like those institutional jailhouse cafeteria knives for him to use." Part of it is education and practice, says Dunia Borga of Alo and La Duni in Dallas. "Since he [son Brandon, age seven] was a little kid, I've taught him to use a kitchen knife. He's got a small knife, like a paring knife, and that's his. He's very careful to put the towel underneath the cutting board so it doesn't slide off."

Other rules for kitchen safety: "Stay away from the fire," says Steve Chiappetti of Viand in Chicago, who hosts a lot of children's cooking classes. "I bought a stove that has the burner knobs on top of the stove, rather than on the side, so the kids couldn't reach it."

Teach your children a healthy respect for kitchen rules. And this is also a good time to start talking about the basics of food safety, why hot foods should stay hot and cold foods cold, for example. And most important: always wash your hands before starting to cook and throughout the preparation process, especially if you are handling raw meats.

"It's Time for a Snack!"

"The prevailing attitude seems to be that children cannot go longer than half an hour without eating. Everywhere my daughter goes, from preschool to library story time to gymnastics class, she is bombarded with sweets, snacks, and 'juice' boxes containing nothing but empty calories."
Kimberly, mother of a three-year-old, in a
Time magazine letter to the editor

When it comes to your preschooler's eating schedule, you will quickly find that many of the adults who lead the activities consider The Snack of the Day to reign supreme. And what I as a mother find so disconcerting about this is that it is usually not even the kids who are asking for these snacks . . . but then again, why would they ever have to, when parents and other adults think it is so important to make food available to them at every turn?

"I was part of a committee helping out with a children's program at my church," one mother told me. "The first thing we had to discuss in planning the event schedule was snack-time: how long would it be, and where would it fit into the day? It's as though the entire session was built around a period for eating."

Sports teams. Nursery school. Sunday school. Story times. Play groups. Music, art, and other classes. Chances are, if your preschooler or older child attends any sort of structured, organized event, there will be "a snack" involved. These snacks run the gamut from nutritious, as in whole fruits or crackers and cheese; to cutesy and silly, like animals or other things made out of foods; to the ridiculously unhealthful, like large iced cupcakes, cookies, or candy. Aside from debating the merits of these many types of snacks, a bigger question that I wish more people would ask is this: why has "the snack" become an expected and required part of every gathering for children?

"I think it's another consequence of an abundance of adult involvement in every aspect of children's activities," one friend told me when we were discussing this, and I fully concur. Kids now go from one organized, scheduled event to the next, often starting as early as their daycare years. All of this structure requires adult supervision and involvement, which leads to adults running the show for kids in the way that they would expect an activity for their own peers to be administered: orderly, with purpose, and according to a timetable. No wasting time. We play for thirty minutes, we read for thirty minutes, we eat for thirty minutes, we have a craft for thirty minutes, and we go home.

End of event. A "snacktime" helps to fill up some of the allotted minutes and can give the adult leaders a few minutes to catch their breaths.

The whole snacking notion is so ingrained in the minds and plans of so many of us that I don't hold out much hope of it changing anytime soon. The best we can hope for, I'm afraid, is that "the snack of the day" will be a relatively healthful one. Many places send home elaborate instructions on providing snacks for children's groups, trying to work around different types of food allergies. Rarely do they recommend avoiding items with high fat, sodium, or sugar content, which can be a hazard to all kids, not just the ones with food allergies. So please do us all a favor and make sure that you send whole fruits or something relatively healthful on the day that you're in charge of your preschooler's class snack!

Skip the Goldfish crackers and cutesy cupcakes in favor of unusual fruits such as papayas, mangoes, or kiwi. Or, better yet, use opportunities like this to introduce your child's schoolmates to something new. Send in samples of three or four different herbs, for example, basil, oregano, cilantro, dill, and mint, along with fruit snacks or vegetables and dip that incorporate or feature these. Preschool teachers are generally most agreeable in allowing such events if a parent takes a little bit of initiative.

I think that one of the major reasons that it's difficult for some parents to stop the excessive snacking at this point in their kids' lives is that it is hard to put a finger on the gradual change in the caloric and eating needs in children as they progress from infant to young toddler, to older toddler, to preschooler and beyond. And there is very little guidance available on this from pediatricians and other health professionals.

Newborns start out needing to eat every two to three hours, which is a lot of feeding, as any new mom can tell you. Months down the line, the number of daily and nightly feedings drops some, and babies may eat slightly more at each feeding session. By early toddlerhood, most kids are on a somewhat regular three-meal-a-day, plus a snack or two, schedule. This is necessary at this age, so that very young kids can fit all of the calories and nutrients that they need into their little stomachs. And of course, at this age, children can't discern "snacking" from "mealtime"; to them, it's all just food, to be consumed whenever it is presented.

But watch Toddler grow; at the age of three or four, she probably doesn't need two snacks a day at all. By now, however, it's become a habit that is hard to break. Throw in the fact that this is the age when many children start to spread their wings and become involved in more of these structured activities, and you have the perfect scenario for endless continued snacking. It's up to the adults in Preschooler's life to guide him to a more standard adult eating schedule, and unfortunately, that's where many of us fail.

Food manufacturers who equate the words "kids" and "snacking" with dollar signs are right in the game, churning out products to fill our "needs" at snacktime. There are so many prepackaged, small-portioned, "kid-friendly" snack food items available at your grocery store that your preschooler could probably happily subsist on these alone. Many are 100-calorie-pack sizes of popular foods. These can serve a good purpose, and they are a handy way for all of us to control portion intake when snacking.

New, too, are products for kids that actually embrace some of the best-known picky eater peeves, says Kristen Harrison, a speech communications professor at the University of Illinois who has studied the effects of television advertising on children. Look at Uncrustables, the frozen snack from Smuckers that (sort of) resembles a peanut butter and jelly sandwich. "They've gone the extra step to remove the crust from the bread, consciously eliminating the part of sandwiches that many kids won't eat," Harrison said. Same with packaged fruits that are already chopped or peeled.

When it comes to your kids and the issue of flavor, keep in mind that all of these processed, prepackaged items are also going to taste sweeter or saltier than whole natural foods such as fruits or homemade goodies. It's always better to snack on the real thing. "We get asked all the time by other parents how we get our daughter to eat peaches and mangoes while her friends at the pool are eating fruit Popsicles," said Pat, the mother of a two-and-a-half-year-old little girl. "The answer is that at home, she just does not have access to anything else, so she literally doesn't know any better." (Or any worse, we should say.)

Snacking vs. "Grazing"

"Lunch is served at different times every day! People eat when they are hungry!"
From "Behind Closed Doors: Brad and Angelina's Nanny Tells All!" *Star* magazine, June 9, 2008

Similar to the concept of snacking is the eating style known in the food business world as "grazing." This refers to the practice of intentionally eating lots of small meals throughout the day, rather than the standard breakfast, lunch, and dinner. A number of parents with whom I talked told me that this is the way their children are accustomed to eating: a little bit of breakfast (maybe), followed by a mid-morning snack, followed by a very small lunch, followed by at least two afternoon snacks whenever they are hungry, followed by a few bites for dinner, and finally something else before going to bed.

Some grazers like to believe that they're onto a healthful eating pattern, but many times this practice differs from "snacking" only in semantics. "Snacks" are supposed to be the chips, candy, or pieces of fruit that we sometimes slip into our diets between meals, to stave off hunger until it's officially time to eat again. "Grazing" implies the planned eating of five, six, or more smaller "meals" throughout the day, all relatively healthful and "meal-like" in their makeup, in place of the more traditional three-times-a-day eating.

The number of grazers is on the rise, according to food marketing analysts, who say that more and more people are now eating unstructured mini-meals throughout the day as part of their "on the go" lifestyles. Although I don't personally care for the concept, I can see how it would appeal to a lot of people, particularly busy professionals. But is grazing a good idea if you're responsible for feeding children, or a family? While there may be some exceptions at certain times, generally, I don't think so.

For one thing, you could never convince me that letting children "graze" throughout the day makes life easier in any way for mom or another caregiver. It's usually enough of an effort to think about three meals a day for my kids; I can't bring myself to even think about having to feed them more often. I guess that when kids are older, they can take on some of this responsibility for themselves, but then you would truly have to keep an eye on what exactly they are eating all day, to make certain that they are getting any semblance of a nutritional diet.

What else is wrong with this? If you're really interested in introducing your children to the idea of "food for flavor," then grazing works against you, as it is another practice that reduces the notion of "enjoying your food" to the level of "consuming something when hungry, just to subsist." If you give your kids a little something to eat every time they tell you they're hungry, instead of teaching them to wait for the next meal, you're essentially saying to them, "There is nothing more important than your immediate hunger, and it's OK to stop whatever it is you are or someone else is doing to satisfy it with anything that you can find."

"I grew up in Europe, where it was three meals a day and that's what you ate," said Chef Marc Murphy of New York's Landmarc restaurant, the father of two young children. "A lot of kids now are always snacking on crap. It's like, there are three meals a day for a reason. Eat the three meals and you'll be fine, and your kids will actually sit down and be hungry and eat what you put in front of them."

From Madison Avenue, with Love

"Fruit snacks and entertainment's favorite characters will join forces, when General Mills introduces an exciting new line-up of Disney-themed fruit snacks. Targeted for kids ages 5–12, the product line will include three permanent SKU's—Winnie the Pooh Fruit Snacks, Mickey Mouse Fruity Peel-Outs, and Disney's Princess Rolls."
From General Mills press release, April 18, 2000

"Over the past few years, Disney has gradually distanced itself from junk food. It ended its McDonald's Happy Meal contract in 2006 and has been expanding its association with healthier foods since then. The result: an abundance of Disney-branded healthy stuff, including fruits, vegetables, and dairy products."
From *Washington Post*, May 3, 2009

When those of us who are now parents were growing up, food companies had their own characters affiliated with their products. Cap'n Crunch, Tony the Tiger, Ronald McDonald, Chef Boyardee . . . you remember those guys. They're still around and, thanks to the powers of advertising and promotion, have made friends with some of your kid's favorite book and cartoon characters. We are now living in a world where SpongeBob SquarePants is selling Popsicles and macaroni and cheese, Spider-Man apparently eats Pop-Tarts, and Barbie stumps for frozen waffles.

Once the sole purview of cereal boxes, tie-ins with television, sports, and movie figures now grace the panels of virtually all food products designed for kids, including cookies and crackers, frozen foods, beverages, snacks, and more.

Marketing and advertising types refer to all of this as "cross-promoting," or "tie-in marketing." These terms refer to the increasingly-popular practice of two or more well-known brands—in most of these cases, a food product and a television, book, or movie figure—joining forces to reach the same target audience—your children! The food product is advertised on the character's television show; the character has his picture splashed on the front of the food product. Kids (the intended audience) react to both. They buy the product, and they watch more of the television show. Everyone is happy.

Most children under the age of about eight can't fully comprehend the concept that commercials and advertising are about selling products. Until they are about six, they usually can't even distinguish television commercials from regular programming. So the use of the friendly characters that young kids see every day on television as product "spokescharacters" on food product packages is a perfect fit. It further blurs the lines between commercial advertising and lovable fantasy friends in already-susceptible little minds.

To get a better handle on exactly how extensive this practice is in the food world, I combed the aisles of several major grocery retailers, closely examining their kids' product selections. What I found was a dizzying array of kids, cartoons, and colors on many different packages, almost all of them on food products that I would not particularly want my children to eat, at least not very often. (Note: it was a dumb idea to take William and Daniel with me when I did this. If you're interested in trying this exercise yourself, do it without your kids in tow!)

Here is a sampling of what I found on the store shelves at the time of this writing.

- The Keebler Elf has teamed with Dora the Explorer to make animal crackers in "5 Dora characters shapes." While Dora is front and center on the box, the Elf is used just in the logo.

- Sesame Street's Big Bird and Ernie and Bert are "spokescharacters" for Apple and Eve Juices.

- Hannah Montana's beaming face is on the front of Danimal smoothies by Dannon Yogurt.

- You'll find a $5 coupon for Hot Wheels or Barbie Sporting Goods in kid's serving-size cans of Chef Boyardee spaghetti and meatballs.

- Yoplait Yogurt features pictures of Blue's Clues, the Backyardagains, and that ubiquitous Dora the Explorer.

- Look for the Berenstain Bears on containers of Hormel Kid's Kitchen products.

- The Flintstones and Curious George are on store brands of fruit-flavored candies.

- More Dora: Campbell's Soup and Unilever's Popsicles.

- Barbie is featured on boxes of Eggo waffles.

- Kraft's Mac & Cheese promotes Spider-Man, Sponge-Bob SquarePants, and Scooby Doo.

And this is an interesting one: General Mills, under the Betty Crocker label, has a line of fruit-flavored snacks featuring Cinderella, Batman, Spider-Man, Tonka Trucks, My Little Pony, the Care Bears, Bugs Bunny, Scooby Doo, and others. These snacks were particularly interesting to me, because of the package design. On the 5¾ inch-by-8¼ inch box (the size of a standard box of cake mix), more than 90% of the front of the box (7½ inches) is devoted to the featured character or toy, with a smattering of candies incorporated into the design. Why, the box looks like it contains a toy, not food! Very clever.

Of all the products that I encountered in my little survey, I came across very few "healthful" products that are supported by some sort of cross-promotional advertising. At the time of this writing, Dora the Explorer could be found on cans of Green Giant sweet corn, Green Giant mixed vegetables, Green Giant frozen green beans with butter sauce, and Green Giant frozen broccoli, corn, and butter sauce. A representative from General Mills, makers of Green Giant products, told me that the character is used as a promotional tie-in to "help parents who struggle to get their kids to eat healthy vegetables."

This may be another indicator that the tide is turning ever so slightly in the right direction. In what is perhaps the biggest step to date in the halt to the blatant association of kiddie characters with unhealthful kiddie foods, in 2006 Disney ended its contract with McDonald's and, the next year, began licensing its characters for use on whole fruits and other "good" foods. Of course the only spot available to advertise on an orange or an apple is on a tiny sticker affixed to the fruit, but still, this was a major turnaround from the traditional thinking that boxes of sugared cereals or bags of fast food were the place to reach kids. The idea has proved so successful for Disney that there are now about 250 offerings available, including such items as the *High School Musical* avocado and Mickey Mouse eggs. Other companies, including Nickelodeon, have vowed to cease all affiliation with unhealthy kid foods.

Much of this is the result of intense pressure from nutrition advocacy groups and government agencies, such as the Federal Trade Commission, which recommended in a 2008 report that "more media and entertainment companies restrict the licensing of their characters to healthier foods and beverages that are marketed to children, so that cross-promotion with popular children's movies and television characters will favor more nutritious foods and drinks." Still, as long as it's working for the companies' bottom lines, we may see more positive changes in the future.

I found study after study confirming that children's behaviors and food preferences were linked directly to the amount of commercials and promotions to which they are exposed. Here's an interesting theory as to why (as if any explanation is needed): Remember the findings of Dr. Leann Birch, who showed that the repeated exposure of young children to new foods can increase acceptability of and preference for those foods, thanks to the familiarity factor? Well, that could apply in some way to product and food exposure via advertising. "While (Birch's) studies have been conducted using direct taste and visual exposure to food, it seems likely that advertising similarly could increase children's familiarity with foods and positively affect food preferences," writes Margo Wooten, PhD, of the Center for Science in the Public Interest, in a report on the widespread effect of advertising food products to children. "Children's liking for foods has been shown to increase after seeing them advertised on television."[53]

Play with Your Food

"All of our items feature great-tasting candy, colorful displays, high perceived value, and lasting play value."
Promotional line from Candyrific's company Web site

So television commercials and their ever-present characters are out to make an impression on children. Not a big deal, you might say, and you'd be partly correct, because these are in fact among the easiest to control. If television programming and its related tie-in marketing becomes too excessive or offensive, all one has to do is turn off the box, and then avoid taking your kids down the relevant aisles at the grocery store. But it's important to note that food sales pitches aimed at kids do not stop there.

It's not much of an overstatement to say that the "marketing to kids" concept has crept into just about every realm of children's lives. To "support and reinforce" (more marketing terms) high-dollar expenditures on television commercials and character licensing agreements, companies are always on the hunt for ways to "leverage the power" of advertising by concocting numerous promotional, public relations, and merchandising programs. These corresponding activities, often referred to as "integrated marketing plans," are in place to "extend the value" of expensive advertising "buys."

And they are everywhere.

How about product placements in toys, games, and books designed for children as young as two or three? A "Froot Loops," or how about an "Oreos," counting book, how cute! In this gem from Nabisco, designed for children as young as age two, "readers [?] can learn to count from one to ten, as each little Oreo cookie is dunked in milk, twisted, stacked, and shared on every page in this study-shaped board book. Full color illustrations!" (Oh, and eat ten cookies along the way. A coupon for Mini Oreos is included with your purchase.) Older kids can learn to "count by fives" with Reese's Pieces or practice adding and division with the *Hershey Kisses Addition Book* and the *Hershey's Milk Chocolate Bar Fractions Book*. Let's set the stage for eating and snacking to be a part of reading and schoolwork! You do the math (so to speak).

What do you get when you combine advertising and games? "Advergames" (another new term for you), and these can be found in abundance on child-focused Web sites, such as Nabiscoworld .com, Candystand.com by Kraft Foods, just-about-any-kids'-cereal-that-you-can-think-of-dot-com, the Coca-Cola "Happiness

Factory" site, and many more. You can buy Coca-Cola infant and toddler clothing, Krispy Kreme toy trucks, Toucan Sam and other icons-of-kids'-cereal stuffed animals, and even a "Barbie Works at McDonald's" restaurant playset. There are kids' clubs supporting kids' products and restaurants of every description, which serve as a convenient mechanism for collecting a database of names and addresses of potential purchasers.

And have you ever noticed that some children's foods exist just as much for play purposes as for eating purposes? This is particularly obvious in the world of confectionary, which features numerous products called "novelty candies" or "interactive candies." Further blurring the line between food and play, you can buy these at both toy stores and in toy departments as well as at places where food is normally sold. Most well-known is probably PEZ, the Austrian company more famous for its dispenser containers than for the actual candy found inside. Beyond that, you can find Etch-a-Sketch lollipops, plastic cell phones with candy, candy fans, all kinds of light-up candy, candy jewelry sets, candy tic tac toe sets and other games, candy lipstick (mirror included) and candy lip gloss, and much more. Many of these feature cartoon and other character tie-ins.

One Plus One Is Two Candy Bars

"Cover Concepts distributes materials, such as textbook covers, coloring books, posters, and other educational materials, free of charge, to over 43,000 public schools, as well as daycare centers, public libraries, and summer camps, reaching a universe of more than 30 million children in grades K–12. Cover Concepts sells advertising space on those materials. Cover Concepts' database enables it to target specific demographic or age groups with branded products and samples."
From *Business Wire* press release, December 2003

Considering all of the activities described above, all of the hoopla that marketing pros whip up to try to separate you from your money and captivate your children's interests and taste buds, the tactic that I personally find the most egregious is the seepage of the advertising and promotional marketing of food products directly into schools and even daycare centers.

A young child's school, some of us still like to think, is a place for learning—about academic subjects and about life. It's where we make friends and memories and play on sports teams and take our first rudimentary steps in society. Increasingly, it is also a place where kids receive regular reminders about the availability of foods that you may prefer that they not eat, often disguised as "learning tools" and in lesson plans. And while a few states do have laws prohibiting various elements of this type of marketing, overall, it is widespread, unregulated, and very welcome in school districts in need of financial support.

You can understand why a food company would love this avenue, for reasons even beyond the sheer number of kids that they reach. Associate your brand and product with "school" and it must be good, pure, and wholesome. The "halo effect," marketers call it, which means that they think that all of the warm fuzzy feelings that kids and their parents associate with taking-an-apple-to-the-teacher will rub off on their product. If The School permits it, it must be fine. What many parents don't realize, however, is that these food (and other) companies are simply taking advantage of many schools' financial shortfalls by offering supplement "educational" products, school supplies, and even cash as a way for strapped school districts to close gaps in budgets. Giving your kids a healthy dose of product messaging along the way is their real aim.

Have you ever had kids—your own or someone else's—ask you to save product box tops or labels from canned goods, to "help out their school"? Very likely, as tens of thousands of schools across the country participate in one or more of these branded programs, designed to provide sporting goods, audio-visual and computer equipment, textbooks, art and music supplies, library books, and other items to cash-strapped school systems. Campbell's Soup alone claims that 80,000 schools and organizations, representing 42 million students, are enrolled in their 30-year-old "Labels for Education" program, which has provided $100 million worth of merchandise to schools. General Mills' "Box Tops for Education" has given $200 million to America's schools in its 11 years.

That's a lot of money, generated by the purchase of a whole lot of soup and cereal and other products, which is, of course, the point. It's also a bit of a paradox, if you think about it, as all of these provided extras could be obtained at lower cost at the retail level. Campbell's, for example, requires the accumulation of 1,350 points in exchange for one copy of a book called *Presidents*. Even if you use only the labels that are worth five points each (many are worth only one point each), a school would have to come up with 270 cans of soup or other Campbell's products. At an average cost of, say, $1.40 per can, that's a very expensive way to procure this book. You can spend $378 on soup, or you can go to a bookstore and get the same book for $19.99. A basketball would "cost" $168; a box of crayons that can easily be found for $2.99 comes to $98. True, these are food products that many families will buy anyway, and it's nice to have something to do with the labels other than throw them away. But with the "gifts" come promotional materials from the companies, including branded logos on posters, screen savers, label and box top collection canisters, and more. They make sure that you never forget the source.

Pizza Hut has a "read-to-me" program for preschoolers ages three to five that rewards them with a personal pan pizza and sticker sheet after they've listened to so many books. There is a "Reading Is Yummy" worksheet that goes along with it, with a place to list the books read on drawings of slices of pizza. And how does one suppose that a three-year-old will get himself to

Pizza Hut to collect this personal pizza? An adult will have to take him there, of course, most likely leading to the purchase of more pizza for other family members. Need an "inspirational speaker" for your class, kindergarten through fifth grade? No problem; just call your local McDonald's "community coordinator" and arrange to have Ronald McDonald himself come to the school. He is available to speak to classes on topics ranging from ecology to safety to reading to character.

And of course, there is direct television advertising into schools, in the form of an enterprise called Channel One. This for-profit company provides electronic equipment such as satellite dishes, wiring, VCRs, and televisions to public and private schools, in exchange for the schools showing their students a 12-minute news program that also happens to contain two minutes of commercials. At this juncture, at least, this is a tool used to reach older kids only; they count six million viewers in over 8,000 middle, junior, and high schools across the country as their audience.

The schools are required by contract to have the programming shown in 80% of the classrooms on 90% of the school days. A corresponding Web site provides classroom materials described as "teachers' tools." Based on a standard 180-day school year, and assuming that Channel One programming is viewed 90% of those days, that amounts to a total of over five hours of commercial programming that each student in a Channel One school receives each year.

Please, Please, Please, Please, Please

"All our advertising is targeted to kids. You want that nag factor so that seven-year-old Sarah is nagging mom in the grocery store to buy Funky Purple ketchup. We're not sure mom would reach out for it on her own."
Senior brand manager at Heinz in a 2001 report

"Some people call it the 'nag factor.' But I see kids as influencers."
Senior Vice President of Digital Media, Cookie Jar Productions,
a producer of children's shows and products

If this short summary on the extent of the marketing of kids' food products has you annoyed, wait until you hear this. In their leave-no-stone-unturned efforts to sell products to your kids, these marketing gurus have gone so far as to devise a method for closing the deal. Actual terms tossed around in these conference rooms: the Nag Factor and Pester Power. Yes, advertisers have discovered that it is most effective to support your children in their attempts to wear you down.

Most of us know from personal experience that we can only take so much nagging from our kids, and of course, our children know that, too. If a parent is inherently opposed to his child having a certain product, it takes an average of nine "asks" from the child before said parent gives in, according to those who have studied this issue.[54] The preteen years are the worst for this; 10% of 12- and 13-year-olds say that they have asked their parents over 50 times to buy them a particular product that they had seen advertised. Manufacturers, advertisers, and even retailers know this, and they do everything they can to constantly remind your kids of what they have for sale. Why do you think children's cereals are positioned on the lower levels of grocery store shelves, for example, or that you can usually find candy and individual sodas waiting for you at the checkout counter?

We parents hate to say "no" all the time. It puts me in a really lousy mood when I constantly have to play bad cop and tell Willie or Daniel, again, that they can't have something that looks appealing. Sometimes I just want to say "yes, of course," and food products, unfortunately, are one of the easiest things to "give in" on. They are relatively inexpensive as compared to such items as electronic or sporting equipment, and can be written off as a just-this-once-treat. Except, of course, they aren't.

Bringing It Back to Taste and Flavor

"48% preferred the McDonald's branded hamburger compared with 37% who preferred the unbranded hamburger."
Results of study on role of branding in influencing children's taste preferences. The hamburgers were identical.

So I hope it is obvious, even from this limited review, that the aggressive promotion of kiddie food products and restaurants is a major force underway in schools, as well as on grocery store shelves, television shows, toys, clothing lines aimed at children, and probably other aspects of kids' worlds.

All of this is to say that you, as parents, are fighting a battle against competitors much more insidious, and with far more dollars at their disposal, than you can imagine. Why do they market in the way that they do? A very simple reason: it works. The food industry collectively spends $1.6 billion annually on advertising budgets for kids' food products, simply because they believe that they're going to see results.[55] And the bottom line numbers are there to prove it: Kellogg's spent $22.2 million just on media advertising and enjoyed a return of $139.8 million in sales of Cheez-It crackers in 2004. McDonald's spent $528.8 million on advertising to reap sales of $24.4 billion the same year.[56]

Food companies are in business to make money by selling their wares. To do that, they must create a consumer demand or fill an existing one for those goods. Advertising, marketing, and all of these promotional gigs do some of each. They convince us that we need certain things for whatever reason, and they tell us how and where to get them. All of this is best accomplished through the use of brands. Apples, for example, aren't branded; they are what is called a "commodity." This means that lots of stores sell them with no name attached, and consumers can get basically the same product from another orchard, another state, or even imported from another country. They offer companies no "added value" because there is no differentiation.

Apples are in many ways the perfect snack food for kids. They come in their own packaging, they are portable because they don't have to be refrigerated, they are nutritious, they are appropriate for just about everybody (apple allergies are unheard of), they taste great, and they are inexpensive to buy. But there is little incentive for major food companies to sell apples "as is," because of the lack of added value. The profit margins are too small.

So to make money on apples, companies have to figure out a way to add something to them that you will pay for. They might look to the convenience factor and sell presliced, prepackaged apples. All of a sudden, to some people, that's worth a little bit more. There is no reason that fast food chains couldn't sell whole apples, but why do that when they can charge you even pennies more to have the apples presliced? And, as a bonus, it reinforces to the consumer the idea that snack foods need to be "packaged" and "processed."

The next step is to take the apples and make something else with them, like apple juice, apple cookies, dried apples, or fruit candies. All of these cost more to produce than simple apples, and that added cost is something that the consumer pays for. And with each step in the process, with each little addition of another ingredient, you're getting farther and farther away from the inherent goodness of the whole apple. Finally, marketers slap a brand name on the sliced apples or the apple juice, cookies, or candies, advertise and promote them to the hilt to create consumer demand, and persuade us that one brand is better than another; and bingo, you have a product that will make its vendor a little money.

Water is another example. Even in the filtered variety, it costs just pennies a gallon and therefore is not a potential money-maker. But put it in a sleek bottle, add some flavoring or vitamins, and you have yourself a "lifestyle product" for which people will pay more.

For evidence as to the effect of all of this, consider a 2007 study in the journal *Pediatrics & Adolescent Medicine*. Here we see some concrete evidence that this intense marketing to kids and its resulting brand awareness of food products do indeed have an impact not only on what kids want to eat, *but on how they come to perceive the flavors and tastes of their food.*

In this fascinating study, California pediatrician Tom Robinson gave 63 children McDonald's hamburgers, chicken nuggets, and French fries, plus store-bought milk or juice and carrots. The children received two samples of each that were identical, one presented in a McDonald's wrapper or cup and the other in plain, unmarked packaging. Dr. Robinson wanted to know whether kids this age—three-and-a-half to about five years old—would perceive any difference in the taste of the foods, based solely on the wrappers and cups.

You can probably guess what happened. Any food from McDonald's apparently tastes better to these kids, even the carrots and beverages that weren't from McDonald's but were served with the Golden Arches logo in view. The labeled french fries were preferred by 77%; 54% opted for the carrots that had the McDonald's label on them. Fewer than 25% of these kids recognized that the food sets tasted the same.[57] "Even the children with the lowest frequency of eating food from McDonald's . . . preferred more of the branded foods," Dr. Robinson wrote in his journal summary.

The power of the brand.

Lest I sound like the biggest stick-in-the-mud you've every heard, let me state that my complaint is not about the individual promotional novelties that these people dream up, the use of cartoon characters in marketing schemes, and all of the individual elements that exist as part of an effective advertising program, *per se*. I can handle the fact that these exist, and even the concepts behind them. I know that it is my job as a parent to make decisions about what to buy and to regulate what my kids eat, just as it is the paid job of the people who work for Hormel and Unilever and ConAgra and others to figure out the best way to sell their products. But what has become unbalanced is the sheer volume of it all. All of this money, all of the research, all of these commercials and new products—it is all there to appeal to the basest desires of young children. No matter how vigilant you are, your kids will eventually find this advertising, or rather, it will find them. As a parent, I feel at times as though I'm trying to stop an avalanche, armed with only a small snow shovel.

In the end, though, I have to believe that simply being aware of the pervasiveness and power of the food marketing world might count for something. If you want to teach your kids about good eating and good food, know and remember that product manufacturers are not always working with you to achieve this goal. Most kiddie food products are all very similar, just packaged differently with an emphasis on individual branding, rather than quality taste and flavor. Nothing makes kids more myopic in their thinking about food than giving them the same thing over and over again. Be aware of this and, while the responsibility to hold the line against such strong influences may be more than many want to accept, at least be cognizant of this direct manipulation and alert to its eventual potential consequences.

All about Beverages

"Is it me, or are there more and more kids drinking Starbucks beverages now? I'm always a little dumbstruck to see a ten-year-old asking her mommy to buy her a vente strawberry and crème frappucino. I cringe

thinking of all the sugar and calories these kids are consuming."
Anna, mom of an eight-year-old and a five-year-old

I treat "beverages" as a separate category in Preschooler's diet, because this is the age that many kids develop flavor preferences that lead to long-term habits regarding what they like to drink. All of those young teens whom you may know who seem to live on soda and sports drinks had to start sometime.

When you think of appropriate beverages for kids in the three- to five-year-old age range, the first thing that comes to mind (I hope) is milk. And the good news is, even though overall consumption of milk is falling and it drops off significantly as children get older, most kids this age do drink their milk. Almost 84% of children under five drink some milk on a given day.[58] The average amount that they consume each day is about a cup and a half, fairly evenly divided between whole milk and lowfat milk. (Only 7% reported drinking skim milk.) According to the Food Guide Pyramid, four- to eight-year-old children need the calcium equivalent of two cups of milk a day.

But children drink about eight cups of fluid a day, so that leaves a lot of room for other beverages. What else are preschoolers drinking?

The slippery slope into the tween and teen world of excessive consumption of sodas, pretty coffee concoctions, highly caffeinated energy drinks, and sports drinks often starts right here. There is a plethora of sweet-tasting, high-in-sugar beverages designed for young kids, available to them, and of course marketed to them, at every turn. From Hi-C to Little Hugs and Capri Sun to Kool-Aid, children consume as many sugary drinks or more as they do 100% fruit juice.[59] More than 10% of the caloric intake in the average child's diet comes from carbonated soft drinks, more than double the amount currently than in 1980. Thirty-nine percent of preschoolers drink soda.[60]

"According to the U.S. Department of Agriculture, even babies consume measurable quantities of soft drinks, and pediatricians say it is not unusual for overweight children to consume 1,200 to 2,000 calories per day from soft drinks," says Marion Nestle, PhD, MPH, in a *New England Journal of Medicine* article. Wow.

"It used to be that children's main beverage was milk," says Pat Harper, registered dietitian and the weight-loss program coordinator at the University of Pittsburgh. "Milk is a very satisfying beverage, providing protein and other nutrients, and a high satiety value, meaning that you feel fuller, longer, after drinking milk.

"But when kids substitute soda pop or lots of juice, they get the same number of calories as milk, but no nutrition and no satiety value. So, a few minutes later, they are hungry again for more food or beverage." This, of course, leads to more eating and drinking, and can quickly lead down the path of too many calories.

Actually, it's very easy to see how all of this can start in the toddler and even baby days, when you look at products like Gerber's "Splashers" purified flavored waters. That's right, now your 18-month-old can has an option for water that is flavored with artificial kiwi, grape, or tropical fruit flavors, and includes 15 grams of sugar per 8-ounce (one-cup) serving. "Oh, that's not *added sugar*," a consumer hotline specialist informs me when I called to ask about this. "It all comes from added juice concentrate." But remember: "juice concentrate" is merely a sweetener, and the end result is the same—sugared water for toddlers. What a perfect way to teach children that water is not worth drinking unless it tastes sweet!

Given the colorful packaging, cartoon character faces on the boxes, and heavy advertising on children's television shows, it would seem as though these fruity, chocolate, and other sweetened beverages must be perfect for kids. The growth in the consumption of sweetened beverages among the under-five set is documented in a recent Columbia University study that showed that kids ages two to five take in an average of 176 calories per day from sugar-sweetened beverages, primarily fruit punches.

"Parents can be easily misled by the labels on fruit punch and sports drink bottles because they make these sugar-sweetened beverages seem essential for good health, when in fact they are nothing more than different forms of sugar water," says Steven Gortmaker, PhD, one of the authors of the report.

This is another instance where vigilance at home may have to compensate for lapses in Preschooler's outside world; you may be surprised at how often these drinks will be made available to your kids during play dates, sports practice sessions, birthday parties, and even school. In a few short years, these youngsters will join the ranks of teens, who now take in an average of 356 calories per day from sodas and other sweetened beverages. Is that the direction you want your preschooler headed in?

Many kids this age are drinking a lot of soda, too, and the concern there is the high caffeine content of the regular drinks. What may be a nice morning jolt for you can be a real hit for Preschooler, as caffeine's effects are dependent on body weight, making it more potent for children. Don't kid yourself: caffeine is a drug, a socially acceptable one, yes, but a substance that tinkers with body chemistry nonetheless. So far, the United States has yet to set guidelines for the amount of caffeine that can be safely consumed by children, but our friends in the Canadian government say no more than 45 milligrams per day for children five and under. That's the equivalent of one 12-ounce can of a typical caffeinated soda, or four 1.5 ounce chocolate bars.

When it comes to soda, remember that 95% of the caffeine is added to the beverages during the manufacturing process. It is *not* a natural component of the product, as it is in, say, coffee or chocolate. Why is it added in the first place? Good question, said Dr. Alan Hirsch, director of the Smell & Taste Treatment and Research Foundation in Chicago. A prolific writer and guest on numerous syndicated television shows, Dr. Hirsch conducts all sorts of interesting studies involving our senses of taste and smell. He recently checked into soda manufacturers' claims that caffeine is added to soft drinks as a "flavoring agent." And he focused on teenagers' ability to discern between caffeinated and noncaffeinated soda, since this age group makes up a large component of that market.

"Caffeine is part of the overall profile of soft drinks," states the American Beverage Association (formerly the National Soft Drink Association) on its Web site. "The bitter taste of caffeine adds to the complex overall flavor profile of soft drinks."

Well, if that's the case, then there should be some discernable difference in the taste of caffeinated and noncaffeinated sodas, right? Hirsch's study found the opposite to be true. "The ability of these teens to tell the difference between regular, fully caffeinated soft drinks and the same soft drink in its noncaffeine version was no better than just a guess," Hirsch told me. In fact, 86% of the teens could not tell the difference between Coca-Cola, Diet Coke, and Pepsi and their caffeine-free equivalents. And yet almost all of these kids said that they normally drink the caffeine version, because they prefer that taste.[61]

As with other drugs, there are side effects when caffeine is consumed in lesser amounts, and, after a period of time, it takes more and more caffeine for the body to receive the desired benefits of alertness and increased concentration. Enter the marketing of soft drinks containing high levels of caffeine, such as Mountain Dew, to adolescent boys via the avenue of "extreme sports," or the rise in sales of caffeine-laden energy drinks such as Red Bull, the fastest growing category of all types of beverages.

Sports drinks, not to be confused with energy drinks, are another beverage category made appealing to children through rampant marketing. Soda manufacturers have voluntarily agreed to drop full-calorie sodas from schools, so they need to find a replacement product. Sports drinks fill the bill, as they can be tied to images of health and exercise. "Essential" for young athletes, says the American Beverage Association. Sports drinks currently account for 20% of beverage sales in schools; in contrast, full-calorie soda has dropped to 29.8%.

"Most kids you see carrying around sports drinks are not athletes," said Mary Story, author of an Institute of Medicine report on the products. "When you look at the ingredients, it's water, high-fructose corn syrup, and salt."

That's the world of beverages that your kids are living in today. Sports drinks represented 2.3% of all beverages consumed in this country in 2005. Wine and spirits together were not even 1.5%. Soft drinks were still king, at 28.3%.

Do your best now, with Preschooler still under your control, to stem the tide of these products. With all of the flashy products available in the category of children's beverages, the venerable duo of plain milk and plain water is still the best choice. (Again, that's *plain* water; lemon, strawberry, and other flavored waters sold on the soft drink shelves are just as unnecessary as those sold in the baby food aisles.) If you do want to play with a little variety, put a slice of fresh lemon, orange, or lime into your kid's cups of water for color and flavor effect. But steer clear of any other enhancements, particularly those of the artificial persuasion.

There is no reason for kids this age (any age, really) to be drinking sodas and many of the other artificial beverages that are designed for them. Milk should not have to taste like strawberries or chocolate for kids to drink it; this is a beverage they've consumed since birth, so "as is" should suffice! Make Kool-Aid and fruit punches off-limits as well. And if you're the leading soda consumer at your house, remember that your actions are speaking volumes to your kids. In a study on the effect of parental role modeling on soda consumption, mothers who drank milk more frequently had five-year-old daughters who drank more milk and substantially fewer soft drinks.[62]

If you can hold all of this in check now, you're that much closer to having the only preteen on the block who isn't hooked on soda.

It All Adds Up to Picky Eating

"Dietary salt is a major determinant of fluid intake in adults; however, little is known about this relationship in children. Sugar-sweetened soft drink consumption is related to childhood obesity, but it is unclear whether there is a link between salt (intake) and sugar-sweetened soft drink consumption."
From *Hypertension*, journal of the American Heart Association

With so much concern about childhood obesity in the health community now, medical science is starting to take a logical next step in research, asking questions that essentially amount to: How do all of these studies tie together? Does excessive consumption of one of the Big Three lead to overconsumption of another? What roles do exercise and genetics play? Are adult-focused studies relevant to young children? And as a culinary professional, I would add another question here: if we can teach our kids to reduce their consumption of the Big Three, will the result be not only a healthier child, but one with a broader palate as well?

English researchers at St. George's University in London found recently that children who eat a low-salt diet drink fewer soft drinks. They went so far as to predict that kids who reduce salt intake by 1 gram each day will also reduce their consumption of soda by 27 grams per day. That was true for all children, ages 4 to 18, regardless of gender, body weight, and level of physical activity.[63] That says to me that there is a clear link between the two.

The link to the sense of flavor and palate development is a less obviously direct one, but it makes sense as well. If you can get Preschooler to reduce his consumption of foods replete with the

Big Three elements, then his diet (and his stomach) will have plenty of room for a broader variety of foods. He will become a more adventuresome eater almost by default.

Yes, I know, again, it's much, much easier said than done. I've learned from this research (and first-hand experience) how pervasive and insidious the Big Three elements are in children's diets and minds, thanks to an almost constant presence in their lives. It remains up to us parents to hold the line, and hold it and hold it, in the face of much opposing pressure. So I encourage you to savor every small victory along the way. A "Hey, Mom, this is really good," said when trying something new and wholesome is your child telling you: "You're doing this right."

What I've Learned

— This is the stage when you can really have some fun with kids and food. Many of them are past the flat-out rejections and table temper tantrums that you may have seen in earlier years, and are beginning to spread their wings in other ways, with new friends, school, and activities. Take advantage of this as a time to expand their food choices as well.

— Cooking with your kids is a great way to open their eyes to the world of food. Even if you're not a cook yourself, and your idea of getting dinner on the table is stopping for takeout, have your children help you as you spoon food onto their plates and talk about what it is that they are eating. Every eating opportunity is a chance for them to learn more about their food, if you take the time to teach them.

— Start paying real attention to the flavors of your own foods. Remember, it all starts with you!

— Snacking and grazing are a way of life for too many kids, and even if you consciously work to keep your kids away from this, they will be influenced by their friends and activities. If snacks are a must, do what you can to make sure that they are healthful and varied as much as possible. Don't allow your kids to fall into the oversnacking or grazing mode at home.

— Snack food companies want your money. They are in business to make money, not to make your children more healthy—that is your job. Their main concern is not so much the healthful properties of their products (or lack thereof), but whether or not you will buy the stuff.

— Allowing the complete insinuation of branded junk and snack foods into schools as a means to sell products is one of the lowest points that we have hit in our public and private education systems. Being vigilant at home is one way to combat this. And don't forget the power of community activism if it's a subject that you feel strongly about.

— As many parents will tell you anecdotally, kids who are picky about one thing tend to be so regarding other foods and beverages as well. For example, if your child will only drink soft drinks or sweetened beverages, she will likely impose a lot of other limitations on her diet. Research is beginning to look at this to determine whether there is a credible link between these actions. I'm willing to go out on a limb now and say that if your child eats too much of one of the Big Three, chances are she's eating too much of the others and not enough of foods that have more nutrients and varied flavors.

CHAPTER 7

⌘

When Problems Start

W hen it comes to raising kids, you may have already noticed that the best of times can quickly become the worst of times.

In the world of foods and eating, it may go something like this: Baby is born and you struggle a bit, but finally get the hang of breast-feeding. Then you decide to wean baby, or baby decides to wean herself, but has problems accepting a bottle. You get the bottle under control and it's time to introduce solids; cereals go well, but other things, maybe not so. Baby decides to teach himself to feed; he practices by dropping foods to the floor and picking up and eating them, using his spoon to apply foods to his hair, gobbling foods one day and refusing them the next.

People remark on how well-behaved your toddler is when dining out; she humbles you by having a total meltdown in a restaurant the next time you eat out. "No" becomes the word most frequently used at the dinner table. The same child who would try anything new, made you so proud by eating Mexican and Thai and Indian food at the age of three, slowly starts crossing foods off of his menu. Within six months, he's down to a steady diet of pizza and peanut butter sandwiches.

In short, just as you are getting used to one stage of eating, it's time for another to begin.

No matter how "good" an eater your child is at any time along the journey, I can promise you that, at some point, problems are going to arise. Whether it's unacceptable behavior at the table, a sudden refusal to eat anything green or without ketchup or mixed together, or a temporary but intense fixation on a few foods, sometime, somewhere, you, too, will be dealing with eating problems in your kids. If they don't approach the level of picky eater, count yourself among the fortunate. But none of us escapes it completely.

In this chapter, I want to address some of the more common eating problems that parents encounter with their young kids, and some practical advice to help you cope. I've collected these ideas primarily from moms and dads who have gone before you, but also from scientific papers and from food professionals. One point to keep in mind about all of these issues: "solving the problem" is not defined as "absolutely no conflict." You may very likely see resistance from your kids, even as you are implementing strategies that they will adapt to, benefit from, and even appreciate in the long run.

Most important, again and always, is consistency and repetition. Trying one solution to a feeding problem one day and then another the next is a recipe for failure. It can be problematic, too, if one parent or caregiver has one standard, and someone else has another that is completely different. To all of the scenarios described here, I would add: to the greatest extent possible, make sure that your spouse, along with any babysitters, nannies, daycare providers, or others who are charged with feeding your child, gets the instructions. Some of these problems are really less about food and eating issues than they are normal children's battles-of-the-will. Do all that you can to make sure that all adults involved are sympathetic to your plan.

"What Is That on That?"

"NO!!! Bean has cheese sauce!"
Evan, age three, commenting on his green bean casserole

Have you ever seen a young child sit at the dinner table and pick apart her meal?

One of the oddest, yet consistent, eating trials that often appear in children this age is a refusal to eat foods that are in any way mixed together. Casseroles, meats with sauces, mixed vegetables, salads, even spaghetti and meat sauce or cereal and milk—dishes that were once eaten happily all of a sudden must be picked apart or even served as separate entities. "But that touched that!" little ones may say, as though the foods have been rendered inedible by the contact. As one exasperated mother put it, "I'm considering threatening to stop cooking altogether, and just feeding him the separate ingredients for every recipe."

It turns out that, according to what little literature actually exists on the subject, this practice may actually stem from another built-in mechanism from Mother Nature. "It's possible that a preference for easily identified foods, eaten separately, enhances the process of food learning," writes Elizabeth Cashdan, PhD, in her paper on children and food acceptance. "Sauces, purees, casseroles, and other mixed prepared foods

obscure a food's identity."[64] Delving further into the anthropo-
logical origin of this, Cashdan writes that it is likely that any
animal would find it adaptive not to eat more than one novel
food at a time, so that the source of any ill effects could be
identified and avoided in the future. Could that be what's
going on here?

Biologically rooted or not, this odd trait can be maddening to
parents, as it prolongs the time it takes to eat a meal and reinforces the image and notion that the child may be a picky eater.
The last thing that many of us want to do is take this child to a
nice restaurant, or someone else's home, and have her completely
dissect the meal. And so many of us turn to a seemingly simple
solution: just give them what they want. Hey, it's not the way I'd
want it, but why not just go ahead and serve pasta with meatballs
in a separate bowl, meats without sauces, or a stratified salad?
You'll find that many children's restaurant menus play right
along with this, offering entrees that are largely unadorned with
anything but the simplest of accompaniments.

The real problem, it seems to me, is that most kids this age
may have very little experience in eating foods in which the
flavors are properly combined, or perhaps they have simply
seen too few variations in flavors. So when they are confronted
with something new, or a new combination, they react by
(a) protesting and (b) resorting to picking through the dish, trying to find, and then focus on, something that is familiar. We
have seen this with our Willie; sometimes when presented with
a new dish that is too complex in flavor combinations for his
mood at the time, he will attempt to break it apart and eat it in
pieces, seeking comfort in familiar flavors. I think that this is fine,
as it is, in fact, most likely just a phase that many preschool-age
kids go through. As long as he eventually tries the entire dish
as part of a complete meal, I try to ignore what's going on here
on his plate.

Interestingly, Cashdan's research shows that the peak time frame for this behavior is the post-toddler stage. In a study of 129 children in which their parents were asked to recall food acceptance patterns, it was at the four-and-a-half-year-old point that most started rejecting the mixed, saucy, or pureed foods they had previously eaten.

Get through this by continuing to offer and provide complete and even complex dishes to kids, even as they are entering this protest zone. If they want to eat it in pieces, OK, but eat it they must. "No, we don't serve this that way," is a perfectly acceptable response to an "I want this without that" demand. Chef Hugo Matheson of Boulder, Colorado's, The Kitchen restaurant, has an interesting solution to this quandary that he sometimes faces with his five-year-old twin sons. "[One of the boys] will say, 'I don't want the sauce, just the pasta.' But if we make it all together, then they actually get quite excited about it. When we were in England, we made pasta and sauce from scratch a few times, and they completely desired it. So when they can associate something with making the whole dish, rather than just having it put in front of them, they get more excited because they've actually had involvement in putting it together."

And speaking of Italian food, several parents told me that pizza is the one food that can sometimes do the trick in getting their kids to try new food combinations. If you have a young child who likes basic tomato-and-cheese pizza—and just about all of them do—try using that as a vehicle to introduce new things. Start with easy-to-like things, such as pineapple chunks and ham slices on a Hawaiian pizza, if you think the going will be rough. Slowly add other items—onions, bacon, different kinds of mushrooms or olives, red and green peppers, and maybe even the dreaded anchovies. You will very likely get some "no ways" along the way, but keep at it as a way of using a familiar food and flavor blend to work through this pick-it-apart stage.

"How Can I Get My Child to Eat Vegetables?"

"My daughter is a wonderful eater. Of course she won't touch vegetables, but what kid does? That part, I consider completely normal."
Hope, mother of a six-year-old girl

"When I was growing up, one of the things my mother used to prepare was canned beets, the ruby red beets that couldn't be more disgusting. I happen to love beets now, but I never got to taste a real beet until I was an adult, so I never knew that I liked beets. So when somebody would offer them to me, I would shy away from them—until I had a fresh candy cane beet that was amazing."
Chef Dan Sachs, Bin 36 Restaurants, Chicago,
father of three children

"My daughter is not a big fan of cooked vegetables like zucchini or broccoli, but she loves spinach salad, even when it is barely dressed. And she will devour grilled onions, cherry tomatoes, sweet potatoes, cucumbers, carrots, jicama, steamed artichokes, and snow peas. So she dislikes cooked broccoli, but she'll eat it raw in a salad. It's a matter of personal taste, and it's the same with her father and me. He loves beets and winter squash and I'm all about eggplant and kale. When she was little, I just kept trying to serve her every vegetable I could find. I think too many parents give up on vegetables the first time broccoli doesn't go over well."
Erin, mother of an 11-year-old

I returned from a local farmer's market one summer day, ready to cook the chard, zucchini, squash, onions, corn, and other goodies that I had found. Since we were soon heading out of town and I knew that nothing would keep for the time we would be away, I decided to serve them all up at once and have a complete veggie dinner that night. "Paul will love this," I thought, as I got to work scrubbing and slicing the produce, giving no thought to the fact that it might be too many vegetables for my little eaters. And sure enough, while he got through the meal, it was not one of Willie's better nights at the table, nor Daniel's either, come to think of it. What was the problem with so many vegetables?

For many kids of all ages, this is the one food category that keeps them from the ranks of being called "good eaters." While many children may be fine with fruits, meats, dairy products, grains, and, of course, anything sweet, throw in something green and that's the end of the line when it comes to eat-all. They pick at it, whine, and put up a good fight, battling the issue of eating vegetables all the way. For other children, it's even worse, and their parents just give up rather than endure the emphatic tantrum.

It's probably little comfort to hear this, but again, there may be some biological element to the reason that so many kids won't eat vegetables. Researcher Elizabeth Cashdan ties a reluctance to eat vegetables to a natural safety factor that keeps young children from attempting to eat poisonous plants. The sharp, bitter taste of many plants prevents primates from eating plant toxins; the same thing may be going on here, Cashdan says. Also, she adds that vegetables have a lower food value compared to meats and fruits, meaning that kids may be predisposed to prefer foods that have a high ratio of calories or protein to fiber since they need those elements for growth.[65]

It's also interesting to note that many vegetables, particularly those with a very sharp taste like spinach, collard greens, and broccoli, may really taste different to young children than they do to adults. Simply put, kids may be better and more sensitive tasters than their parents are, because children have up to 10,000 taste buds, compared to less than half that for adults. Our taste buds diminish in number as we age, making the strong cauliflower, chard, or cheese more palatable to you than it would be to your toddler or preschooler.

All of this is to say that you're not alone if you have a child who refuses to eat vegetables—hopefully, it is a natural phase that she will outgrow. The problem comes when parents just accept this as the way it must be and stop presenting vegetables as a part of the meal. This prevents any exposure to the variety of flavors and nutrients that vegetables bring to our diets, and will reinforce in the child's mind that he doesn't like their taste. So keep at it, probably not as zealously as I tried to do with an insistence on an all-vegetable dinner, but slowly, one zucchini, one eggplant, one asparagus serving at a time.

"(My son) loves vegetables," says Chef Zak Pelaccio of New York's Fatty Crab and Five Ninth Restaurants, speaking of his five-year-old. "I get him to eat them by cooking the vegetables properly, and that includes flavoring with a bit of salt. People are so afraid of salt, even used in fine cooking, where it is essential, and yet they eat processed foods. They have no idea how much sodium is in processed foods."

And Chicagoan Steve Chiappetti, chef at Viand, adds this about his six- and three-year-olds: "The texture (of vegetables) is very important—nothing stringy, nothing that's going to make them gag. Celery, I didn't even approach until my daughter was about five, because there are so many strings in it. Carrots, I always blanch or cook to the point where they're tender, so they're not crisp and mealy in the mouth. It's such a textural thing with them."

Talk to your kids about how much you like certain vegetables, and take them with you to the grocery store or farmer's market so they can see the variety. And as Chef Pelaccio says, pay attention to the way they are prepared, tasting them for flavor as they cook. If you're steaming things like sliced zucchini, carrots, or spinach or cooking them in the microwave, add a little chopped garlic or grated fresh ginger to the water. Try cooking them in different ways; grilled vegetables are particularly tasty and can be sampled on a restaurant outing if too difficult to prepare at home. Roast root vegetables, such as turnips, beets, and parsnips, as well as the dreaded Brussels sprouts, with a little bit of olive oil, salt, and pepper, and you may be surprised at the reaction you get.

Many people (like grandparents, perhaps) will suggest adding flavor to cooked vegetables in the form of fats, such as salad dressing, excessive butter, or melted cheeses. "My kids are great about eating their broccoli," boasted one mom, who casually added that the only way they'd ever had it was drowned in Velveeta. Does this "count" toward vegetable consumption? Of course it does, as the nutrients are still there along with the added calories, but proceed carefully, as it may set a bad precedent that causes other problems down the road. The last thing that you want your kids thinking is that broccoli or any other vegetable must be submerged in cheese, butter, or another fat to be palatable. I think it's a matter of finding balance: a little bit of ranch salad dressing on crudités, for example, may be a way of enticing children to try raw sliced vegetables. Broccoli casserole—another way of coating the vegetable with fat—may be a better introduction than steamed broccoli. But try to keep the variety factor top of mind. There are many, many ways to prepare, serve, and eat vegetables; some may taste better to kids than others, but in the end, it is the taste and flavor of the fresh vegetable that they should learn to recognize.

And when your little one does finally dare to sample a new vegetable? Try not to make too big of a deal out of it, no matter how things go. If she actually likes the carrots or broccoli and agrees to eat an additional bite or two, don't trip all over yourself with the praise and the "Good job!" accolades. It's hard to resist, I know, because you feel like you might actually be making a tiny step forward in the right direction, but too much attention to the outcome is counterproductive. In the same way, try to shrug off even a serious negative reaction with an "OK, we'll try that again on another day." (Just be sure to really do that!) The eventual goal is to have your kids learn to recognize and accept vegetables as just another food choice, one that we happily and willingly include in our diets, in whatever form they may be presented.

A Hot Dog by Any Other Name

"Mommy! Ice cream!"
Two-year-old's comment when seeing a bowl of mashed potatoes

"Who wants a hot dog?" yelled the grill master at a recent cookout my family attended, watching the little kids at the party swarm to him like ants. Paper plates in hand, they lined up to get toasted buns and grilled dogs, to be coated with spicy mustard, ketchup, and relish. So many takers, in fact, that the hot dogs ran out before little Jackson reached the front of the line.

Not a problem, his father thought, reaching with the tongs to put a sausage on Jackson's plate. Dad then helped him doctor it up to perfection and sat down with him at the picnic table to eat. "Wow, this is the biggest hot dog I've ever seen!" Jackson said with delight as he picked up the roll to eat.

"Oh, you got a kielbasa!" responded one well-meaning mom. "Yes, those are delicious, too."

The smile faded. Down went the bun, without even a bite being taken. "A *what?*" Jackson said. And of course, that was the end of that. No amount of coaxing could convince this five-year-old to just try the kielbasa, which looked and smelled almost exactly like a hot dog. "It's even better than a hot dog," his dad said, trying hard to rescue the situation. "Kielbasa is a little spicy and has a kick to it that you don't get in hot dogs." No sale. The kielbasa was passed along to another lucky partygoer, leaving Jackson to settle for a lunch-meat sandwich.

What happened here? Was merely the unfamiliar name of the food alone enough to discourage a sampling? Apparently so. When it comes to kids, the mere name by which a food is referred to can sometimes be enough to earn it a thumbs down.

I was talking to another friend recently whose young daughter has turned into a picky eater. All of a sudden, he says, she has decided that she likes chicken, but not pork or most other meats. Since this newfound preference has come out of the blue, it's causing problems with such things as barbecue and even hamburgers. "And so," my friend told me conspiratorially, "we just tell her that everything is chicken."

Now, I suppose that's one way to handle the problem. But in the end, is this really the best idea, for you or for your child? What if someone else calls you on it, as happened to Jackson's dad at the picnic? What happens when your child figures out on her own that you've been fibbing? You may have a long-term eating strike on your hands, adding to a sense of food confusion.

Of course, this can also work in the reverse: sometimes a catchy or amusing name will persuade a reluctant taster to give it a try. My chef friends seem to be particularly creative about this as a way to get their own kids to eat well, or to try new foods. Maybe it comes from all of that experience in writing menus. Hugo Matheson of The Kitchen in Boulder, Colorado, brews up a Magic Yogurt for his five-year-old twins, which he says is a combination of regular yogurt and maple syrup, honey, or jam. Jeff and Barbara Black, both chefs and owners of Black Salt in Washington, D.C., say that their eight-year-old loves Magic Soup, which is basically a homemade chicken-and-vegetable soup with a little rice or pasta. I guess chefs do work magic in the kitchen, after all.

Two great things about having young children: you know that you are smarter than they are (for the time being, at least), and that they will believe just about anything you say. Of course, this also involves a big responsibility, as you are establishing a trust factor that may last for many years. But if you start early enough, you can use all of this in your favor when it comes to food. Be *positive* in your tone of voice and attitude when presenting something with an unfamiliar name to your kids. Get them to giggle about it, if it's a silly or funny-sounding name, always reinforcing the idea that *it will taste great!*

My personal belief is that any attempt to trick your child into eating one thing by telling her it's another is a bad idea, no better than the deception of sneaking pureed vegetables into her desserts. So much of it comes down to issues of trust with food. Remember that besides nutrients and satiation, you are giving your kids emotional messages with the food that you serve. To do so under false pretenses tells them that Mom and Dad don't respect their ability to handle something unfamiliar and that you care more about getting them to do what you want them to do than you do about honoring their opinions and feelings.

There is nothing wrong with a child sincerely not liking kielbasa or pork or anything, as long as he tries it and realizes that there may be times when he will have to eat it. But to try to manipulate him by pretending that it's something else puts a parent on shaky ground. Instead, go back to the message of variety and "things taste different, but they are all good in their own way." And repeat. Again, and again, and again, as necessary.

"Sit Down!"

"My sister and her three-year-old were visiting recently. Mia (the child) never stopped playing to eat, never even came to the table. My sister just followed her around the house with forkfuls of

food, trying to pop something into her mouth whenever she could.
It made me crazy just to watch it."
Liz, mother of a six-year-old and a one-year-old

My fear is that Willie will one day choose for my epitaph two words that he hears every day from me: *Sit Down!*

Several years ago, I visited some friends who at the time had four children under the age of six living in their home. To say that mealtime was disorganized would be a huge understatement. It was more like a four-ring circus, with little individual acts going on at the same time. But even more striking to me was the evidence left behind from the attempts made to get these kids to eat. All over the house (and I mean everywhere), there were half-eaten containers of yogurt, open packages of cheese, dried-up grape stems with two or three grapes remaining, half-slices of pizza, and sandwiches with a couple of bites gone. The message was obvious, at least to me: why *should* these kids ever stop playing long enough to eat a meal? All they had to do was walk (or run or crawl) ten feet, and they would find something else to munch on.

When you combine an energetic kid with food that may not be particularly pleasing to him, an appetite that fluctuates, and any number of interesting distractions, it can all add up to chaos at mealtime. Up and down, in and out of the chair, running around the room, "but I have to do this first"—it's enough to set any parent on edge. So up you go, chasing him around with a spoonful of food, trying to catch him on the fly for a quick swallow. It's bad enough when this happens at home, but at least, you reason, you can handle it here. Then you go to someone else's house for dinner, have the grandparents over for a meal, or try to venture out to a restaurant, and you realize from the cold stares that you get that things really may be out of control. How did this happen?

Take solace in the fact that just about every child goes through this stage at some point. So anyone who has ever had children can, in some small way, sympathize with you, although a lot of people seem to have selective memories about how much of this they had to deal with from their own kids. (Do try to keep that in mind when you're in public and the recipient of judgmental looks from older people. They've just forgotten.) The trick for you now is how you handle it, minimizing the level of disruption whenever possible and encouraging your child to move past this stage as quickly as possible, to more acceptable table behavior.

It helps to keep your expectations realistic. Most two- or three-year-olds are simply not ready to endure a lengthy sitting session, be it for mealtime or anything else. Small victories are important here, and progress is measured incrementally. Junior sat still while Mom and Dad ate a salad *and* an entrée at the restaurant; terrific! Little One finished everything on her plate without getting up once tonight; good girl! Maybe a little treat, such as a family walk around the block or an extra story, is in order.

By the time kids hit the preschool years, however, "mealtime" should have some concrete meaning to them, and describe a definite time and place in their day. This is another example of how you may have to rethink your own habits and adjust your schedule to fit your kids' needs. If *you* are used to eating on the fly, start making a real effort to sit down and spend a little time with your food. Eating while standing over the kitchen sink, next to the microwave, or in the TV room with your feet propped up is not the example you want to set. Give yourself a definite amount of time—even ten minutes is good, if that's all you can spare—to *sit down* at the *table* to eat. Everyone else can be instructed, and expected, to follow suit.

One time that will almost certainly be a problem, however, even if your children are otherwise pretty good on this issue, is group gatherings, especially new situations, that involve a lot of other kids. It is at times like these that you will see that many other parents don't exactly impose the "sit down" rule in their own homes. Depending on how swept up in the moment your child is, or how much of a leader/follower she feels like being, you are witness to a side of your child that you normally don't experience. This has happened to us on a number of occasions: getting Willie to sit down and eat at home or at restaurants or when he's around one other child or two is usually no problem, but change the setting to a birthday party, family reunion, large Thanksgiving dinner, or something else that involves a lot of young guests, and even if he's hungry and wants to eat, he'll participate in the uproar.

My philosophy is to not make a big deal about this, recognize it for what it is, and brace myself for the next day or so, when he may exhibit fallout behavior from not enough sleep and too little food. This is another example of the "we don't do this at home" mindset. It's OK for him to enjoy the people and the party and the fun; for kids, it's rarely about the food, anyway. But as a daily way of life? No.

"Sit down" should mean just that. It also means "stay seated," until you have finished all that you want to eat. When you do get up to start another activity, this meal is officially over. There is no coming back a half hour later for another few bites, no reheating food after the cartoon is over or another round of "Chutes and Ladders" is complete. This will take some work and rework on your end, Mom and Dad, but it is an important issue on which to stand firm.

And by the way, this lesson can start early. The first couple of times that Baby Daniel tried to stand up in his high chair brought a couple of chuckles, as in "oh, no, we have a *climber!*" But that had to stop, obviously, for safety reasons and also to begin to teach him the rule: we sit down to eat. When we stand up and try to leave the table, that's it for the meal.

"Will You Please Hurry Up and Finish Eating?"

"Will you PLEASE hurry up and finish eating?"
Me to Willie, on many occasions

Does this scene sound familiar? You sit down at the table, you eat your dinner, chatting a bit with whomever is there. You may have seconds or a small dessert or glass of wine, all the while trying to coax the little ones around you to keep up the pace on their eating. You finish your meal, you're ready to get up, clean up, and get on with whatever you have to do that evening—except for the fact that one child or more is still sitting there, giggling, talking about everything and nothing, pushing peas around on his plate, and, in general just dragging out the whole meal experience.

So many mothers and fathers have told me that their patience wears thin at the dinner table, as they wait for their young children to finish their meals. These are the nights that don't necessarily result in total meltdowns, or even a refusal to eventually eat the food, but just seem to take forever to get through the eating process. Believe me, I know first-hand how exasperating this can be, although I'm not sure why we so often single out mealtime as the worst example of kids' procrastination. It seems to me that children this age like to prolong just about everything that they do!

I wish that I had a great solution for you on this one, but I'm afraid that I'm in the same boat that many of you are. Little Daniel is really starting to test us on this one, as he'll often want to eat a few bites of his lunch or dinner, get up from the table to do something else, and then come back to it minutes or even hours later, still picking away a bite at a time. He's experimented, too, with trying to take his dish into other rooms of the house, all the while eating just enough to encourage us to let him remain in control of the timetable.

The converse of all of this is, I suppose, equally unappealing, as I really don't want my boys rushing through their meals, stuffing food into their mouths as they dash off to their next activity. So I'm learning that the key to teaching timing and pacing with eating is to set the tone that mealtimes are an event unto themselves. By that I mean, try to set aside a certain amount of time to eat, even if it's just 10 or 15 minutes, rather than allowing meals to happen on the fly. It's become too easy to take breakfast with us in the car on the way to school, or to eat lunch at our desks while working, or to try to cram in dinner between soccer practice, evening meetings, and homework. This sends everyone the message that eating is the least important thing that we do, and that food is merely our fuel to keep us burning through other activities.

If all family members take a designated time to sit down at the table, preferably together, to consume a meal, it helps to solidify in young children's minds the idea that now is the time to be eating. We eat breakfast before we go to school or to daycare. We eat our lunch before we go outside or take a nap. Dinner has a start time and an end time. Eventually, young children will realize that they need to keep up the pace; Daddy is getting up to wash the dishes and Mommy is going to help Older Brother with homework, so I'd better finish eating, too. I can't promise that this will happen immediately, or that you won't have some testy sessions along the way, but keep at it. A set structure does a lot to instill this desired behavior.

Another version of this problem that we run into with Willie from time to time is his immediate acceptance and eating of one item on his plate, along with a refusal to eat anything else. He'll want seconds, thirds, even more of one favorite item, while leaving everything else untouched, in effect dragging out the meal with the hopes that he can fill up on what he wants and leave the rest. The obvious answer might be to just go with what he's eating and let him have all he wants, but we try not to fall into that hole. I think it's important for kids at least by preschool age to begin to understand the vision of *meals*, how they are put together, and why certain dishes are chosen to complement each other. This is an important concept for kids to learn in their understanding of not only the nutritional components of what they eat, but also the flavor value.

To teach them to eat the entire dinner, you begin as you always do, by putting an appropriate, child-size serving of each item onto your kids' plates. What to say when they want more meat and potatoes, but won't even try the corn or beans or salad? Stand firm on this one, and say "No. Not until you've tried everything else on your plate."

"But . . . but, I don't *lllllliiiiikkkkkkkeeeee* that." And so it goes. It's time to move on, in your head and in your words, to the title of the next section.

"I Am Not a Short-Order Cook"

"I am not kidding when I say that my neighbor runs her house like a restaurant. She has three kids, plus a husband, and all of them like different things. So she'll start with something basic, like chicken, and fry it for one person, bake it with sauce for another, stir-fry it for someone else. I have no idea what she eats. I can't decide if this woman is a super-mom or just plain crazy."
Celia, mother of a five-year-old and a two-year-old

"When I was growing up, my mom had a refrigerator magnet that read: 'Tonight's Dinner. Two Choices: Take It or Leave It.'"
Jennifer, mom-to-be

In talking to numerous mothers of young children as research for this book, I was amazed at how many rely on some version of this statement to effectively run their households. It's a line worth committing to memory and sealing in that book of Greatest Mommy Lines Ever. Repeat after me: I Am Not a Short-Order Cook!

If you can make this your mantra, I can promise that you'll go a long way, quickly, down the road toward the goal of producing a child who will eat just about anything.

Of course, you actually have to stick to this mantra in practice and make it an absolute rule of the kitchen, one that you never, and I mean never, break. As soon as you start making even minor exceptions, as in "but she's the baby," or "will something else make you feel better after your bad day at school?" or "OK, what *will* you eat?" you've lost major ground.

Note that this is not at all the same thing as refusing to let your children express what they would like to have for lunch or dinner, or keeping them out of the meal decision process completely. Far from it; everyone in the family, I believe, should have a chance to offer an appropriate level of input, and have known favorites and recipe requests. But there has to be a reasonable balance, and that doesn't mean a fifty-fifty split. The cook, the parents, the host, the caregiver, the responsible adult gets the lion's share of the vote in deciding what will be served. I'm a firm believer that on this issue, the kids are along for the ride.

This means that if you decide to have baked chicken, rice, peas, and salad for dinner, everyone in the family partakes of baked chicken, rice, peas, and salad. You don't have to justify that decision; it can be because it's the easiest thing for you to make, because you have the ingredients in the freezer, or because you've found a new recipe that you want to try. Or maybe, it's just what you are in the mood for that day. Assuming that you are providing a variety of nutritious and relatively interesting meals on a rotating basis, then I say, Chef Rules when it comes to the final decision on what to have on any given night.

And if the little ones at the table protest? Even the American Academy of Pediatrics backs up the hard-line approach, saying "Don't be afraid to let the child go hungry if he or she won't eat what is served. Which is worse, an occasional missed meal or a parent who is a perpetual short-order cook?" Indeed.

"I made a quick pasta and vegetable dish for my kids before my husband and I went out to dinner one night," my friend Sandy told me. "And I left complete instructions with the babysitter on how to reheat it and when to give it to them. But when we got home, the pasta was in the refrigerator and there was a half-eaten bowl of scrambled eggs beside the stove. 'But that's what Pete wanted,' the babysitter said." That explanation reminded me that an essential factor in maintaining your credibility with this rule is making sure that anyone else who watches your kids at least knows how you feel about this issue.

I Am Not a Short-Order Cook.

I Am Not a Short-Order Cook.

Repeat, as needed, to yourself and your kids. Eventually, they may get the message.

"And I Am Not a Waitress"

"I've let my kids get into some really bad habits at the dinner table, and one of them is letting them get up after their meals without helping to clear the table. I hate the idea that I wait on them hand and foot, but that's what it feels like sometimes. How did I get put in charge of all of this?"
Laura, mother of a six-year-old, nine-year-old, twelve-year-old, and fourteen-year-old

In the same way that I repeat the line "I Am Not a Short-Order Cook" to my Willie, I also add the line "I Am Not a Waitress." What does this mean? It means that children at toddler and preschool age and above can and should be expected to help get their food on the table, as well as clean up after themselves.

Since about the time that he turned three, every time we eat at home, we ask Willie to go to the cupboard and "get your placemat" before eating a meal. As he's grown older, we've added simple tasks to this process; he is now responsible for bringing his own dishes to the table ("Use two hands!"), as well as his own napkin, cup, and fork or spoon. After he's finished eating, before he can do anything else, Willie is reminded and required to "take dishes to the kitchen." And yes, we have to repeat this at just about every meal, sometimes to great resistance. At the moment, he is fascinated with the process of how the dishwasher should be loaded. I am not above milking that for all it's worth.

This is also a good time to remind young children that they should "thank the chef," or whomever prepared their meal, for the nice dinner. A bit self-serving in our case, I suppose, as that person is most often *moi*, but I do think it's a good habit to get into. Mealtimes are all about rituals, and this is a nice one to add.

And as with everything else, repetition and more repetition is the key to success. This is one of those wonderful skills that your kids may use to surprise you at a very opportune time, as when they are visiting at your mother-in-law's house and they carry their dishes to the kitchen after dinner without being told to do so. Or if you're at the company family picnic and, in front of your co-workers (and hopefully your boss), they pick up their trash and dispose of it properly. People will fall over themselves asking how you "get your kids to behave so well." Practice, practice, practice!

"Ew, Gross, Yuck, Disgusting"

"Eccchhh! What are you trying to do to me, Mom?"
(canned "audience" laughter)
Brilliant line from smart-alec kid on a television sitcom

"I picked up my son and two of his friends from school on St. Patrick's Day and mentioned in the car that I had made Irish stew and soda bread for dinner that night," one of my friends, the mother of a six-year-old boy, told me. "Probably to impress his friends, he started making gagging noises and carrying on about wanting to run away from home and eat at McDonald's every night. When we got home, I sat him down and told him that he is never, ever to carry on like that about food or meals. Food may be a lot of things, but in this house it is never terrible, disgusting, gross, or any other derogatory word that little boys, especially, can come up with."

You tell him, mom. Kids may say the darndest things, but there is something wrong, I think, in letting them make excessively negative comments about their food. Besides being highly annoying, it displays a blatant lack of respect for and understanding of all of the effort that went into getting that food to them, not to mention how fortunate they are to have something to eat in the first place.

I think that a lot of everyday eating problems are solved as children grow to develop an appreciation for their food and the work that it takes to produce it. It is not something to be taken for granted. It's easy to see how kids fall into that mindset, however, by just walking into your average American grocery store. The abundance of foods and choices available looks overwhelming. Of course, the natural inclination is to think that this is the way it is everywhere, for everyone. But food should not be treated as a given.

Teach your kids that someone—as in, you and/or your spouse—had to work to earn the money to buy the food that they eat every day. Farmers had to grow it; processors had to produce it; wholesalers and truckers brought it to them; retailers had to put it on the shelves. Someone—again, guess who?—has to give thought to what they should eat, go to the grocery store or a restaurant and purchase it, and get it to them. Most food that they eat has to be prepared in some way, whether simply reheated or thawed, or made into an elaborate dish. Whether the preparation involves hours or minutes of your time is irrelevant; it is all done in your kids' best interest and should be afforded respect accordingly.

The other point to consider about the "yuck" factor is a psychological one, as negative statements like this often become self-fulfilling prophesies. Once a child's vocabulary in describing his food is allowed to slide to this point, it's very difficult to turn around the mindset and convince her that she will indeed enjoy the meal. One friend told me that her two-year-old nephew prefaces every bite of food that he takes with a grimace and a shrill "ewwwwwwwwwwwww," simply because that is what he's always heard his older brother do. "And then he goes along and happily eats the food," she adds. "I guess he just thinks that this is what you're supposed to say when food is placed in front of you."

I continue to marvel that one of the great advantages of dealing with children this age is that they are (generally) so adaptable to any idea that is presented to them. When things go wrong in children's lives, we speak of how resilient they are in rebounding from unhappy situations. So, put this power-of-positive thinking to work when it comes to teaching them about food. Staying positive in descriptions of food, and requiring them to do the same, is an important step in that process.

Not surprisingly, this is an area about which the chefs whom I interviewed for this book felt very strongly. Because they are in the service industry themselves and are constantly judged and rated on how they prepare meals for other people, many of them are very sensitive to the blunt and sometimes nasty comments that children may make about their food. When he takes his five- and two-and-a-half-year-old children to restaurants, for example, Chef Robbie Lewis of San Francisco's Bacar restaurant makes it a point to talk to his kids about how they are to act and respond to the food that they receive. "They know that Daddy's in the business," he said. "'These people are in Daddy's business and we want to look good,' I'll say. 'You don't want people to come into Daddy's restaurant and trash it, do you? So let's be good to these people.'

"We also talk to [my five-year-old] about trying things, and not wasting food," Lewis continued. "Food is hard to come by and a lot of people work very hard to grow it. And a lot of people in this world don't have the option of throwing food away. So we put some social awareness on him, to be responsible for not wasting food. Not that I make him eat crap he doesn't want to eat, but I at least would like for him to try things."

Chef Frank Bonnano of Luca d'Italia and Mizuna in Denver says that his wife has worked to teach his six- and four-year-old sons the value of their food. "[My wife] is very good at that," Bonnano said. "She makes them appreciate what food is—that it's something you don't just go to the store and pick up without a lot of thought. There is a lot of work and effort and expense that went into it.

"She always says to them, 'That's what Daddy does for a living. He cooks for a living for us. His job is to use dead animals and turn them into food. And to kid ourselves that the food just shows up on the shelves would be silly.'"

And this from Chef Hugo Matheson of Boulder, Colorado's The Kitchen: "My idea is to get them [his five-year-old twins] to respect food, not waste food, and try and appreciate it for what it is, a precious commodity, really. It's a big battle judging exactly what you need to buy. With the kids in restaurants, I'm always saying, 'eat this first and then if you need more, we'll see.'"

Several years ago, before we had children, Paul and I hosted a dinner party at our house for several couples, one of whom brought along their teenage daughter. We had gone to a lot of trouble to prepare a nice meal, and while I would never pretend that the results were chef-quality, they were certainly tasty and attractive enough. This teen, however, was having none of it. All through dinner, she carried on with dramatic sighs and shakes of her head, professing that she "couldn't eat any of this" and leaving no doubt by the expressions on her face as to her opinion of the meal. I'm not sure which annoyed me more: the idea that she was so coddled that she wasn't expected to behave better in the home of her parents' friends, or that she was obviously allowed to express any opinion she cared to about food that someone else had prepared for her. Either way, it's something I had better not ever hear from my boys!

What Happened to Number Two?

"Liza (age 7) will be fine with anything, anywhere, but if you decide to go for something other than pizza, let me know, because I'll have to pack something special for Lynne (age 5)."
Message on a mom's voice mail, as she attempted to make birthday party plans for her daughter

So you're raising a great little eater, one who loves Indian food and green vegetables and octopus and will try any new dish that is put before him. "We must be doing something right," you smugly think, "I mean, I should write a book about this." Then little brother or sister comes along and you look forward to another adventurous diner joining your table. Except it doesn't exactly work out that way.

"My *older* son/daughter is the best eater!" so many, many parents told me. "We thought we had this child eating everything in the bag. Then Baby Ethan/Emily/Ian/Isabel came along and we got a dose of reality."

Yes, there is nothing quite as humbling to second-time-around parents as realizing that, for whatever reason, Number Two is not going to follow the script. Here you are, finally professional, experienced parents who know exactly what to do, and you find that you have on your hands a new customer who didn't read the playbook. You may see this in many areas of your kids' personalities as they grow up, but if you're like me, one of the areas where you will notice it first is in how they eat and learn about food. Our Baby Daniel fit right in. From birth, he's been a voracious eater (unlike Willie, who didn't really impress with the volume of food he consumed, especially as a baby), but there are times that he seems "pickier" about likes and dislikes. "What in the world is going on here?" I have often asked.

Well, a lot of it is us. Daniel is a different child, of course, but Paul and I are also different parents to him than we were to Willie when he was a firstborn, only child. I'm the first to say that it's easier to slip a little on your own rules and policies with the second and subsequent children than it is with your oldest. For one thing, you may not have the time, not to mention the energy and stamina, to watch things quite so closely. And you've seen in your first child that a few slipups here and there are not the end of the world.

This can be treacherous thinking, however, if you let it go too far and end up giving Number Two too many passes. Just because "we" may have moved on to the older-child eating stage, doesn't mean that he has. Daniel still needs the same level of exposure to new foods, the same level of repetition in introducing new things, the same table training that Willie received. We often have to remind ourselves that Daniel is three years younger and that it's not fair to compare his actions to his older brother's, or to have the same expectations of him that we do now of Willie.

Of course, there are some benefits to being the younger brother. Daniel has his own role model to emulate, and often will try something new simply because Willie is eating it. Lately, he's been insisting on using a small fork rather than a spoon to eat his meals, just to be more like everyone else. He's figured out the difference between the containers of whole milk (his milk) and skim milk (everyone else's milk) in the refrigerator, and starts a sippy-cup strike if he is served something other than what Willie drinks. The desire to keep up, at least at this point, is very strong.

So don't write off the younger kids. Instead, to the greatest extent possible, include them in the meal routine at the family table. You may find yourself needing an extra dose of patience to handle their normal, age-appropriate feeding quirks, especially if you've already invested a lot in your older child's food knowledge. "I thought we were past that!" you may find yourself wistfully thinking. And you will be again, soon enough. Remember, your firstborn didn't become the "good eater" that she is today by accident.

Daniel's bad scenes in restaurants, his boycotts of certain foods, the endless dragging out of meals—we had all of those nights with Willie, too. I think we've just blissfully forgotten.

When the Problem Is Really Serious

Every now and then—not often, fortunately—there comes a child who has very serious problems in learning to eat. Many of these kids start out in the 1% or 2% of all infants who have such severe feeding problems that they end up malnourished; 70% of those infants will still have food problems at ages four to six.[66] There are medical terms such as "infantile anorexia," "feeding disorder of state regulation," "sensory food aversions," and "post-traumatic feeding disorder" that describe the heartbreaking conditions of babies and young children who are the most seriously afflicted.

Some of those kids end up under the care of such doctors as Irene Chatoor, a psychiatrist at the Children's National Medical Center in Washington, D.C., who specializes in treating children with severe feeding disorders. Chatoor's 2001 paper describing diagnosis and treatment of the most serious eating and feeding disorders in young children provides guidance in identifying those who may need professional intervention. This is important even beyond the obvious nutritional issues. A later study led by Chatoor found that toddlers determined to be "healthy eaters" had significantly higher scores on the Mental Development Index (MDI) than did toddlers who were classified as either picky eaters or suffering from infantile anorexia.[67]

The first to use the term "infantile anorexia," Dr. Chatoor writes that this disorder usually becomes apparent when a child is between six months and three years of age, as the transitions between spoon- and self-feeding are occurring. This is a child who simply refuses to eat adequate amounts of food for at least one month, preferring to explore, climb, play, or interact with others rather than eat. There is usually no sign that this child is ever hungry. Parents, as a result, often become very frustrated and try to regulate the child's food intake by any method they can think of: coaxing, distracting, force-feeding, threatening, feeding the kid while he is playing or trying to sleep, or offering any number of foods, just to get some calories down. This, in turn, creates a vicious cycle as the child is actually hampered from learning what it means to be "hungry," and instead has to rely increasingly on these external actions to "tell him" when he needs to eat. Treatment for infantile anorexia may involve some form of therapy to help the parents redirect the child's attention during mealtime to help him focus on his food and become aware of internal hunger signals.

When first introduced to baby or table foods, some infants exhibit what Chatoor calls sensory food aversions. These toddlers may come across as the ultimate Picky Eaters, refusing to eat certain foods because of their smell, taste, texture, or appearance. They are quite happy, however, to eat foods of their liking. As we've discussed already, this is actually a quite common occurrence in young kids and reaches feeding disorder status only if the food aversions result in nutritional deficiencies or other problems. Parental guidance is sometimes needed to remedy extremes of this condition, as are vitamins and other food supplements to maintain nutrient intake.

Chatoor also writes about newborns who have a difficult time learning to feed because they either can't calm themselves down enough, or can't wake up and become alert enough, to take in the milk. There are also medical conditions in babies such as reflux and food allergies that prevent or hamper the development of proper feeding skills. Post-traumatic feeding disorder, according to Chatoor, is a condition in which infants who cannot communicate verbally have a real fear of eating food or drinking from a bottle after an episode of choking or severe gagging. Each of these requires medical intervention to solve the problem.

Many other books have been written about children who display such picky eater traits that their health and emotional well-being may be jeopardized. Some of these provide information and strategies that may be helpful in dealing with these problems. If you or your pediatrician suspects that your child may fall into this category, I urge you to seek advanced nutritional and medical guidance as soon as possible, to begin intervention and therapy at as young an age as possible. These problems can be remedied, but they may require behavior modification actions administered as advised by a healthcare professional.

What I've Learned

— Consistency and repetition are the two best guidelines for any actions taken to remedy picky eating problems that may (will) arise. Often, it doesn't matter so much exactly what you choose to do as it matters that you pick one solution and make sure that everyone involved in feeding your child follows it.

— Almost all children, even your star eaters, will go through weird food phases, picky eater stages, and days/weeks/months when they practically battle with you about their food. *Continue to serve it as it should be served* through as much of this as you possibly can, allowing them to choose to eat it in the way that they prefer. Eventually—sometimes, very eventually—this behavior should wane, to be replaced by a new acceptance of the foods.

— When it comes to things that are really important that they learn to eat, like vegetables, keep serving them, even in the face of seemingly endless rejection. Try to serve in new ways, in new dishes, and in new incarnations, if you can, but stop short of trickery. Actually hiding vegetables in other foods or disguising them as something else will eventually backfire on you.

— If you're having a hard time getting your kids to stop what they're doing and come to the table to eat, work to make mealtime more structured. Depending on your child's age and how far this problem has spun out of control, you may have to employ some real discipline techniques to establish a new Mealtime Is Mealtime rule. This is one area of childrearing, however, where I can promise you that the extra time spent on this issue will be well worth it.

— If you have the opposite problem and your child seems to linger at the table, dragging out his mealtime far past everyone else's, you also need to step in and firm up the schedule. A very matter-of-fact "finish your dinner and then it will be time for your story," or "time to play with your trucks," may do the trick. The key, again, is not to pay special attention or play the reward, but merely the next step in the evening's schedule.

— *Never* get into the habit of cooking a special meal or food for your child, asking him if he'd "rather have something else," or doing anything that in any way supports manipulative actions to agree to eat.

— Teaching kids to respect food is a key step toward teaching them to love it.

— There are some feeding problems that go beyond the scope of the "taste" issue. If you suspect that your child's eating or feeding problems are causing serious health or emotional problems, take up the problem with your pediatrician.

CHAPTER 8

⌘

Chefs Speak: Practicing What They Preach

Chefs, particularly those of the "celebrity" variety, are the de facto Arbiters of Taste in the minds of many Americans. We watch them on television, flock to their restaurants, devour their cookbooks, and generally regard any comments they make on foods and food trends to be absolute fact. Not a bad position to be in for the few who make it to the very top, usually after years of culinary school, the subsequent training, and hours upon hours of grueling, late-night and weekend kitchen work. Celebrity Chef status brings additional responsibilities of promotional tours, high-risk business dealings, and the expectation of empire building. It's no wonder that this lifestyle takes a toll on the family lives of many in the profession, yet a surprising number of chefs do manage to maintain some semblance of "normalcy" in this area. And for many, that includes children.

In my work with restaurant chefs from around the country, I often speak to them about their children and the issue of developing young palates. Almost without exception, this is a topic that they feel passionately about, as they want their own offspring to learn from an early age how to appreciate and discern good food. Who could be a better source of advice on this topic than chefs themselves, I thought?

So, as part of my research for this book on how children's palates are developed, I sought out and talked to a lot of chefs. I looked for chefs who represent a variety of ethnic cuisines, and who come from a broad geographic mix. I spoke to men and women and to top star chefs with nationally known names and to a few who are just starting out, or who are best known in their region. My one requirement was that they had to have children of their own and at least some responsibility for feeding them.

Just as in speaking to any group of parents, I ran into a wide range of opinions on some of the hot eating topics, but there were a lot of consistencies as well. Most revealing: these professional foodies overwhelmingly said that yes, they care very much about what their kids eat and that they eventually learn to appreciate food. For the most part, they are trying to make an effort to teach their kids a love for good food. But thanks to harried work schedules, a need for convenience, and the parental uncertainty that hits us all from time to time, many chefs admitted that they have a hard time modeling this "eat good food" behavior for their own children, even though they take a lot of pleasure in providing it for others. So you see, while they may have a knowledge level about food and flavor that we lack, most of these chefs are not really very different from the rest of us.

When I asked my chef friends whether their children are "good eaters," I got a lot of "yes, but" types of answers, as in "yes, she was at one point, but now she's giving us some problems," or "yes, for the most part, as long as it's not anything weird." If this sounds familiar, read on; some of these chefs have come up with creative solutions to help their kids get through picky eater phases.

A Fine Palate: Is It Born or Bred?

"We have dinner at the restaurant every night because Dad is working and we want to have dinner with him, a family dinner. It's kind of hard having a restaurant where a child can come in and order whatever he wants. Monday is our day off and we're home. There, I don't cook separately for him. And when we're at home, this is what's for dinner."
Chef Dunia Borga, pastry chef at La Duni and Alo Restaurants, Dallas, and mom to a seven-year-old

Few kids have it so good. Imagine being able to walk into a top restaurant pretty much any time, wander through the kitchen, and pick whatever looks good to eat, or to have a superstar-caliber chef living in your own home whose responsibility is to keep you well-fed. It would be a nice life, wouldn't it?

Yet, kids being kids, they don't always see it that way.

For one thing, chefs' children, like most other kids, appear to be very concerned about what they are eating in comparison to their friends. This makes them not always appreciative, shall we say, of the high quality of food that they get at home. Like kids everywhere, they are not immune to peer pressure, especially if they have friends who eat more typical children's fare. So if that means passing up the grilled fish or homemade roasted chicken in favor of macaroni and cheese or pizza from a box, well, sometimes they're more than happy to do that. Dunia and Taco Borga, chef owners of La Duni and Alo, favorite Latin spots in Dallas, report that their seven-year-old son used to eat everything but, more recently, has become a problem eater.

"We ate everything, and we gave him everything to eat [when he was little]," Dunia says. "But once he started school, I think it was peer pressure, because his friends were not eating what he was eating, so he changed 100%. All of a sudden, he came home and he wouldn't eat anything colored—it was just potatoes and meat. He comes home and asks me for things that I don't buy, that we don't normally eat, but he's seen them on TV or one of his friends gave it to him."

Monica Bhide, a cookbook author, cooking instructor, and expert on Indian cuisine, agreed, saying about her nine-year-old son, "He used to try everything, but his friends would be like 'Ew, you eat spinach,' or 'Ew, you eat sushi?' So he stopped eating interesting things for awhile because he used to get so upset. I wanted him to continue his good eating without feeling bad about it, so I took him to a sushi-making class for kids, just to show him that there are other people his age who do enjoy different foods, and that it's OK to do so. I think that made a huge difference. I'm hoping he's getting over all of this as he gets older."

The major boost that chefs' kids seem to have over other children is the constant positive vibes that they get about food. In their households, food is fun; it's an adventure; it's a way of life. Many of the chefs spoke passionately about taking their kids to farmer's markets or to the grocery store, starting little gardens with them, or inviting them to be in the kitchen at their restaurant. "We take our boys to the farmer's market and let them taste the fruits," said John Stehling, chef and owner of Early Girl Eatery in Asheville, North Carolina, of his two young sons. "Now, they only like certain things but I know their palates will grow." Fred Neuville's Fat Hen Restaurant on John's Island, South Carolina, uses produce grown by children at a nearby Montessori school.

Gayle Pirie and husband, John Clark, of Foreign Cinema in San Francisco, host their child's class at the restaurant, as do Barbara and Jeff Black of Black Salt Restaurant in Washington, D.C. John Brand of Las Canarias in San Antonio hosts cooking classes for the friends of his three young boys, many of whom had no interest in what they were eating until they started hanging around his sons. "And we talk a lot about food," adds Chef Robbie Lewis of San Francisco's Bacar Restaurant. "I think it helps to get kids thinking about what they are eating."

Chicago chef and restaurateur Dan Sachs effuses about the role that food plays in his three children's lives: "Good food is part of our life. It's what they know. We went strawberry picking and the strawberries weren't the most exciting part to my kids, it was the fresh peas that they grow there. So we bought a bunch of peas and came back and shelled them, and [made] this orzo and pea and tomato thing. It was the whole experience—they were eating the peas raw—that makes kids love food. It's what I love, too.

"And all of a sudden, what they know of peas becomes a delicious flavor memory, and they're going to be pea-eaters for their whole lives. But if you grew up on Jolly Green Giant frozen peas and that's what you know, why would you want to be a good green food eater?"

Emphatically, I also heard this: firm voices when it comes to the question of whether or not the kids are expected to eat what their parents eat. "I don't cook separately for him," Dunia Borga told me about her seven-year-old, echoing the comments made by many others. "In a large family, we don't have the time to cater to each one of their cravings, so they are forced to conform to a certain degree," said New Orleans' John Besh, chef at Restaurant August, of his four sons.

"You're gonna eat what Mommy and Daddy are eating," Frank Bonnano, chef at Denver's Luca d'Italia, tells his six- and four-year-old boys. "And then when they go to bed and say, 'Daddy, I'm hungry,' I say, well, you should have eaten your broccoli—then you wouldn't be hungry." Gayle Pirie and John Clark have the same idea when it comes to meals for their nine- and three-year-olds, stating, "If they don't want to eat it, they don't eat it, and then they go to bed hungry. That's just the better way. We don't make them a whole new dinner; that backfires. It just teaches them to do that again, and then they'll reject the second dinner as well."

"I think there is something wrong with giving (kids) too much choice," adds Hugo Matheson, chef at The Kitchen in Boulder, Colorado. "I won't say 'What do you want for breakfast?' I'll just put the cereal on the table and say, 'Here's breakfast.' And they (his five-year-old twins) don't argue with it. Whereas if you give them a choice—do you want toast, do you want bacon— then they get sort of confused. That's one of the big issues, and I think it's the downfall of them just getting on and eating."

In the end, does all of this lead to "better" eating among chefs' kids than among their friends?

"Definitely," Dan Sachs responded. "Their friends' eating habits are more straightforward; they're not as willing to try. They won't even eat fish, let alone mussels. But these are also the kids that are getting peanut butter and jelly five days a week." Most of the other chefs whom I talked to agreed that it at least seems this way to them. "How can you allow your kid to go without eating fruit?" asks Chef Gary Donlick of Atlanta's Pano's and Paul's. "But I see that in my daughter's friends." "I would say his friends eat very mild foods and they're not very adventurous," said Monica Bhide. "If there is a kid who eats kebabs, he'll eat only chicken kebabs. Or if he eats plain white rice, he won't try brown rice."

"It's so easy, I guess, to grab those Lunchables and say, 'Here you go,'" adds Steve Chiappetti, chef at Chicago's Viand restaurant. "But even though it's easy to send a kid off with that, it takes the work out of it. That's not us."

Thanks, But No Thanks

"If they're with a babysitter or something, I'm not going to be
over-regimented about it. I think it's all about finding a balance.
There are some days we'll stop off—about once a year—and
get a burger and fries."
Chef Hugo Matheson, The Kitchen, Boulder, Colorado

In this quest to produce good little eaters, are there any foods that chefs consider completely off the menu for their kids?

Most of these chefs keep a pretty tight handle on their kids' diets, and if they do list forbidden items, it's generally the things that you would expect to see: a lot of candy, fast food. Juice, again, is often mentioned as a "no." But there are exceptions, sometimes, even to the hard and fast rules.

"Soda. We don't have soda in our house," adds Gayle Pirie. "They can have a soda, but it's very rare. They eat cookies and stuff and I don't hide candy. I let them have it, not all the time, but it's not forbidden. I just don't want them to grow up wanting it because they've never had it. If you give your kid a Happy Meal once a week when they're little, they get addicted to that for sure. They get addicted to the salt and the convenience and the toy, and all that. If you don't do it, they don't crave it, they don't grow up making it a part of their lives."

"Well, they are exposed to [fast food]," says Frank Bonnano of his boys. "The grandparents come, and when the grandparents come, if they want to take the kids to McDonald's, well, you know, you can't deny Mamma and Pop-Pop. So that's when they get it."

"To sound like Northern California radish-lovers, we don't do a lot of fast food or processed food," Robbie Lewis responded. "And it's also how San Francisco is built. San Francisco is not harboring a bunch of fast food restaurants in very convenient places. Almost all of the fast food restaurants are on the periphery of the city[; it's] not even possible to drive into [such] situations. I grew up in Arkansas, so I grew up eating fast food and frozen pizzas and Pop-Tarts. But to me, now, it's not easy to get that fast food here. In Little Rock, it's on every block."

What's in That Brown Bag?

"I've had more than one teacher comment on [my son's] lunches.
His lunches are a derivative of leftovers from the night before.
I think that was after a day when I sent him to school with
some lamb chops and steamed artichokes; the teachers
commented on his 'aggressive' lunch menu."
Chef Robbie Lewis, Bacar restaurant, San Francisco

It must be more of that peer pressure of kids eating around other kids, because on the issue of school and snacking and lunches, chefs gave me some very mixed answers. "The more unusual, the better!" some seemed to say, keeping up their performance cooking even as it goes into plastic bags and lunch pails. "Keep it simple, it's not that important," was the other side of this coin, with just as many chefs saying that their kids eat and snack on the same thing that your kids do at school every day.

"[School lunch is] one thing we don't fool around with too much; it's a matter of not being the unusual kid on the block," says Chicago's Steve Chiappetti. "It's PB&J and things like that for school. We stick to the norm. We don't want [our six-year-old daughter] to be in school and have people say, 'what is *that?*' We want her to eat."

But in Berkeley, California, where Chefs Gayle Pirie and John Clark send their child to a public school, it's a different story. "I fix a sandwich, and a little treat or an organic apple," she says, when asked about school lunches. "There's no soda allowed at his school; you can't bring a soda for lunch. Fast food isn't allowed at the school, either. It's not like that in the whole country, but it is here in Berkeley. They say, 'make a healthy choice for your lunch,' and it's great."

Dan Sachs of Chicago's Bin 36 puts in the effort to make sure that lunch for his three children is a healthful and well-rounded part of their food for the day. "It's a pain in the butt to do that as a parent, to have creative lunches and all of that, but for better or worse, I don't give them the same lunch every day. I want them to be excited about what they are having," he says. "Sometimes it's more junky and sometimes it's more healthy; I try to be balanced about it. They're always curious about and excited about what lunch is on any given day. And it's all the little things that get kids excited about food.

"[I know that] I have a huge advantage because I have a food background and my kids are in the restaurants all the time, so they are curious about it naturally. But that said, I see what other people give their kids to eat for school lunches, and then they wonder why they won't try new things."

Welcome to My Restaurant: What We Wish Parents Knew

"We took a family trip to Italy, where eating with your kids is sort of the way of life and not a big deal. We went to this really nice restaurant (mistakenly) for lunch, where they required a jacket, and they let me borrow one. But it was so natural for them to include our kids. They had special china for children; it was just how they do business there. Versus here, where it's like, 'Oh my God, the kids!'"
Dan Sachs, Chicago restaurateur and father of three children

When it comes to dining out with children in tow, many chefs can speak to both sides of the coin. They know what it's like to set the stage for a nice evening for their guests, only to have a screaming toddler disrupt things for everyone. But chefs are parents, too, and many of them can feel your pain. Sometimes, they're even the ones in that situation.

"We've walked out of restaurants with them kicking and screaming," confesses Frank Bonnano of his two little boys. "With our order in, I've dropped the credit card and said, 'We're leaving.' Same thing in the grocery store. You could have a basket full of groceries and if they melt down over that thing they want, we leave."

"I've had to pick him up and walk out," says Chef Dunia Burgo of Alo and La Duni in Dallas, of her now seven-year-old son. "I'm not going to put up with [misbehaving in restaurants]. I'm very sensitive to it, maybe because I have restaurants, and I want to make sure everybody else around me is enjoying their meal and is not bothered."

"We take them out to restaurants and sometimes you win and sometimes you lose," Gayle Pirie added. "My nine-year-old is a breeze; he'll go anywhere. Our three-year-old is difficult, and she's been difficult to go out with for about a year. And we get stressed out at restaurants if she's being bad. It's very stressful on mom and dad if a child is not behaving. But we don't want to shelter them and limit their experiences, because then as they get older, they're less adaptable. But you do pay a price if they're not well-behaved."

So how best to handle temper tantrums and meltdowns in restaurants, if yours happens to be the problem child? Unanimous agreement: deal with it, Mom and Dad, and fast. Don't just ignore the situation.

"What we've always done with our kids is just pick them up, bring them into the bathroom, and have a talk with them," says Chef Marc Murphy. "Remove them from the situation and remove them from driving everybody else crazy. If that doesn't work, take them home. I don't think there is any reason to make everyone else suffer. But you do see parents whose kids are throwing a fit and they're like, 'Oh, well,' and they just kind of ignore it. I'm thinking, 'Are you kidding me? You're not the only one here!'"

"I think everyone in the restaurant business has seen situations where parents are not mindful of their child throwing things all over the place, making a total disruptive mess," says Chef Richard Vellante of Legal Seafoods in Boston, who has a young son and a daughter. "The parents should not overstep their bounds. The waiter is not there to babysit the child, and sometimes, that does happen. I've seen parents that don't even know the child is walking around the restaurant or making a huge mess."

If your kids are causing a problem, "You can't be afraid to say, 'Your behavior is not conducive to us being out tonight, and it's time for us to leave,'" Vellante continued. "It's almost like when you make a deal with someone, you can't be afraid to get up and walk away from the deal. Sometimes a walk outside, getting them away from the atmosphere, will help. But I haven't been above just saying, 'It's time for us to go.' It doesn't happen too often, but I've been there."

Most of these chefs, though, hasten to add that they welcome children, even very young children, at their establishments and go out of their way to help out parents. "We have about 25 high chairs at Landmarc and sometimes they're all being used," says Marc Murphy. "I've made it uber-clear to my service staff that they are here to make every family with children that comes in feel extremely comfortable," said Chef Robbie Lewis.

"I've told them that many parents are nervous that their kid's going to act up, and there's a really finite timeline before kids start to wig out. So I say, 'Get the order in fast, ask if they'd like a certain food early, don't screw around, don't give them the usual, let me come back and take your drink order line.' Just get them what they need, fast, because they don't have a lot of time."

And quite a few pointed out that many adults have no right to a superior attitude about kids in restaurants, as they—the adults—are sometimes the worst offenders on the behavior front. "Oh, yeah, late at night you have the adults who are the worst anyway," Murphy continued. "They get drunk and knock stuff over." Dan Sachs in Chicago says that it's typically "parents, unencumbered for the evening by children and out for a partying good time," who are the most poorly behaved. "There's an occasional super-bad kid," Sachs says, "but there are far more poorly behaved adults."

Chefs also shared success stories about nights out on the town with their kids. Chef Cathal Armstrong of Alexandria, Virginia's Restaurant Eve took his eight- and five-year-olds to dinner at posh Restaurant Boulud in New York, during the Christmas holiday rush season, no less, and with a 9:00 p.m. dinner reservation. "The whole place was agape when they walked in," Armstrong told me. "I mean, we got stares from everyone in the restaurant. But they behaved beautifully and sat through six appetizers, four entrées and seven desserts. Actually, they behaved better than some of the adults."

Dunia and Taco Borga, chefs in Dallas, took their son to elegant York Street when he was about four. "And he sat and had a marvelous dinner," Borga remembers. "We always look at the menu and see what he likes, and we might ask them to put sauce on the side, or something like that. The only place I've ever had a problem with that is in France. We were in Paris with him and we asked for sauce on the side, and the French just don't do that. That's the way it comes, and I'm sorry. After about the second day, he was fine with it."

Well-behaved children are often well-rewarded in many top restaurants, with such prizes as special tours of the restaurant, extra goodies on a dessert plate, or a chance to go to the kitchen to make their own dessert. Chef Bob Carter of Charleston, South

Carolina's Peninsula Grill enjoys going out to tables that have young children, wearing a tall chef's hat and inviting them back to the kitchen for a make-your-own sundae treat. "The parents love this, because it gives them a few minutes' break to enjoy their dessert and wine," he said.

So bring them on, most chefs say, your kids really are very welcome. Many go out of their way to make children feel at home, often at the direction of top management. Boston's Legal Seafoods chef Richard Vellante's own two children made suggestions as to what these establishments should provide for kids; they helped design interactive questions for parents and kids, things like "Have you ever gone fishing?" or "Have you ever eaten a lobster?" Marc Murphy gives all of his young visitors free cotton candy at the end of the meal, with their parents' permission. Chef Frank Bonnano gives out pizza dough at Osteria in Denver; kids can use it to make their own shapes. He then takes it back into the kitchen and bakes it for them.

All of this is designed to make not only the kids happy, but parents feel comfortable in bringing their kids around. Says New Orleans chef John Besh: "I want families to be at peace bringing children to our restaurants, because if they feel comfortable doing so, we'll build a future generation of diners."

And for the Children This Evening?

That said, if you do take your kids out to eat at a nice place, these chefs would love to see them eat. Really eat, real food. Chef Marc Collins of Circa 1886 in Charleston, South Carolina, says that often people will call ahead and say things like, "Make sure you have chicken nuggets available tonight; I'm bringing my children." Despite this, many chefs prefer to work with you to provide a smaller sampling of something on the regular menu, at a reduced price, so that your kids can get the full restaurant experience. Children's meals out don't always have to be fish sticks and spaghetti.

When asked about what things on their menus are the most popular with kids, chefs mentioned petit steak filets, grilled salmon, and housemade pastas. Chef Hugo Matheson has kids who "die for duck confit" or specialty versions of typical children's fare, like burrata cheese on toast with anchovies, what he calls "the ultimate grilled cheese sandwich." Steve Chiappetti's Viand restaurant in Chicago has a "junk food dessert cart" that he says kids all love. "It has a homemade version of Twinkies and Oreos: two chocolate egg-white cookies with an Italian buttercream between them."

Gayle Pirie sees two kinds of kid diners at her Foreign Cinema restaurant in San Francisco, almost two extremes. "It's odd," she says. "[Some] order quail or risotto. And then I'll get a table full of teenagers who are 18 years old, and they all want the kids' menu. They've never been outside of their box, and they're afraid it's going to be [terrible] because they've never eaten it. And I tell them, 'no, it's the opposite. You've never tried anything, so you have this fear.'"

Still, there are signs that children's menus are one area in which we food-lovers will see some progress. A recent food-service industry report claims that more and more children's menus are including items typically found on adult menus—smaller portions of premium steaks, fresh fish, and baked or grilled chicken, along with vegetables and fruits. They report a growing preference (among kids) for bolder, spicier flavors, such as teriyaki, chili, and chipotle.

"Kids today are growing up with a wider range of cuisine and restaurant options than ever before, and are growing more adventurous than previous generations," adds Sheila Weiss, a consultant to the National Restaurant Association. "Ethnic food is growing in popularity among young diners, and many are trying things like pad Thai, Peruvian-style chicken, and other dishes typically not thought of as kids' favorites."[68]

But for now, at least, these are the exception, as young children still say that pasta and French fries are their favorite dishes in full-service restaurants.[69] So in my personal view, what I've stated earlier in this book bears repeating: just stay away from traditional kid's menus altogether, and you'll already be one step ahead. Your kids never even have to know that kiddie options even exist. Put yourself, and your children, into the hands of the chef at the restaurant you've chosen. Take the advice of Chef Marc Collins and "order what you want, and split it all with the kids." Go for the experience, and you'll all gain from it.

Food writer David Kamp's *New York Times* Dining Out section piece, "Don't Point That Menu at My Child, Please," summarizes all of this beautifully, telling the story of his realization that too many children and their parents rely on kiddie foods, at the expense of developing more mature tastes. It seems that in his salad days as a parent, he was a big fan of children's menus, thinking it was a great thing that "children at good restaurants could now be immediately placated with children's food, so that we adults could plunge worry-free into our adult business of drinking alcohol and eating things with tentacles."

But, in all of his dining adventures with his wife and two kids, he slowly began to see things in a new light. After his kids ordered chicken fingers with fries "for about the 102nd or 103rd time," he writes, "I came to the realization that America is in the grips of a nefarious chicken-finger pandemic, in which a blandly tasty foodstuff has somehow become the de facto official nibble of our young." Further singing my song, Kamp goes on to state that while the health implications of this are obvious, "I'm much more rankled by its palate-deadening potential. Far from being advanced, the standard children's menu is regressive, encouraging children (and their misguided parents) to believe that there is a rigidly delineated 'kid's cuisine' that exists entirely apart from grown-up cuisine."

I couldn't have said it better myself.

What I've Learned

— On the whole, the children of chefs do seem to be better eaters, with more varied diets and broader palates, than your average kid.

— Having said that, these children are not in any way special breeds, with super genes that make them automatically more accepting of a wider range of foods than other kids their age. What they seem to have that most other kids lack is constant exposure to new foods, an inherent interest in their homes in trying new things, and the influence of at least one adult who has a passion for food.

— Many chefs view issues concerning their children's eating habits through the lens of discipline—the same regimented discipline that they bring to their kitchens everyday. They expect from their kids a sense of respect for food and the processes that bring it to us. They instill that in their children by insisting on such points as good manners at the table, a willingness to try new things, and a refusal to be wasteful.

— Without going crazy about it, most chefs keep an eye on what their young children eat, severely curtailing exposure to foods and beverages that they don't want them to have.

— At the same time, most chefs know that their kids live in a world where their food values are not the norm. They want their children to learn and to "rise above," but also to fit into their environment.

— They really, really don't mind if you bring your kids to their very nice restaurant, as long as you are in full control of the situation. In fact, most of them are very glad to see the kids with you.

— They love it when your kids order or eat something off of the adult menu. They'll make that spaghetti alfredo or hot dog if they must, but they are truly delighted when a young soul experiences and enjoys their fine cooking.

CHAPTER 9

⌘

Restaurant Dining

*"Well, if Jake will only eat pizza and Abigail doesn't do hamburgers
and you promised Luke Mexican, where can we go for lunch?"*
Mom chit-chat overheard at neighborhood swimming club

Because of our professions, my husband and I eat out a lot in
restaurants. (It's a tough assignment, I know.) Sometimes when
we're lucky, these restaurants are the top-of-the line places that
feature nationally known chefs and stellar food, or perhaps wonderful little hidden jewels that focus on the cuisine of a specific
region or ethnicity. More often, especially these days, they may
be casual neighborhood-type spots, where the food may not be
outstanding, but it is reliably very good.

When William and then Daniel were born, we knew we'd have to slow down a bit in our restaurant research, but in no way could we or did we want to stop altogether. And as they've grown, it's actually gotten a little easier, not harder, to include them at the table. But that doesn't stop the stares and rolled eyes that sometimes come from other diners when we appear at the front door, holding the hand of a young child and carrying an infant.

"Oh, Great, Here Come Some People with a Kid!"

"We went out for dinner to a neighborhood place with our one-year-old, and the whole experience was a disaster with her screeching and banging her sippy cup on the table nonstop. We have hardly ever gone out with the baby, precisely for this reason. We took her right after she ate her own dinner at home so she would be full, brought snacks and toys, but nothing calmed her. What are we doing wrong??"
Post on parenting Web site

Oh, dear.

Who among us can't feel for these people? Even if the situation wasn't as distracting for those around them as they might have feared, it's enough of a bad memory that these parents most likely will think long and hard before trying such a venture again. When you're the one in this situation, it's easy to imagine that this is the worst it's ever been, and that no child has ever misbehaved as badly in a restaurant as yours just did.

When we take Willie and Daniel out to nice restaurants, I'm always impressed by the sheer graciousness that the restaurant staff shows us. No matter where we have been, they always at least act delighted to welcome our kids as fellow diners. I can't think of one example where we've been made to feel like they were out of place, no matter the location or rating of the restaurant. Granted, there have been times when we have been shown to the worst table in the house (in the back, near the kitchen, beside the bathrooms) when others were clearly available, but never has it been stated or even implied to us that young children are not welcome. Perhaps this has given us a false sense of courage or entitlement, but my rule is this: if the restaurant has a high chair or booster seat on their premises, then ours are not the first children to darken their doorways. (We have only encountered a couple of instances where neither of these was available, and we discovered that stacked telephone books work just fine.) And so we boldly proceed. Just smile at or ignore the people at the next table who may appear to have other opinions.

I will also tell you up front that I do not mean to imply that all of our restaurant visits have gone well. We have definitely had some less-than-perfect (really embarrassing) evenings in nice restaurants. (Incidents in Asheville, North Carolina, and Honolulu, Hawaii, immediately come to mind and still make me cringe.) And I hasten to add that if either of the boys ever becomes the slightest problem, one of us takes the said offender out of the restaurant pronto, and goes to the car or the lobby, until either the upset child is able to calm down or the other person can get the remains of dinner packed to go and paid for. Needless to say, times like these do not make pleasant memories, but under no circumstances should a child be permitted to disrupt other diners or impair the enjoyment of their meal. But, thankfully, those nights were and are much more the exception than the rule.

They can take a long time to live down in your own mind, however, and I can see why many parents who have young children, or even just one little one, are hesitant about eating out more often, especially when it comes to venturing into new restaurants, or places that are more upscale. But I do think it's important to try, and try often, even if you have to really force yourself to go. It's a little bit like exercising on a regular basis: you might hate the thought of it, and it takes discipline to commit to a regular regime, but once you do, it eventually becomes incorporated into your life and you do it without much thought.

One of the most important reasons that it's worthwhile to make an effort to eat out with young children is for the practice, for both them and you. Your years of dining out with little kids may not bring the best gastronomic experiences of your life, but they shouldn't be viewed through that lens. The ultimate goal at this point, it seems to me, is to train your young kids to grow up to be the ten- or twelve-year-olds whom you can take anywhere to eat and who know how to make table conversation and have at least a passing interest in food. So many parents have told me that having these skills in place at a young age is helpful in navigating the uncertain waters that may come in the teen and later years. Believe it or not, it can all start here.

For now, remember this: it really helps to lower your expectations a bit. If your baby, toddler, preschooler, or even older child is with you, you simply are not going to have the same dining experience that you did before they entered the picture. This is not to say that it is a worse experience (not always, anyway), but simply different. You most likely cannot spend 20 minutes chatting over a cocktail before you even look at the menu, peruse the specials as if your dinner entrée choice is the most important decision you will make all day, or linger endlessly over coffee after dessert. In fact, the first time or two you do this, you may be surprised to compare the 45 minutes that you spend just getting yourselves out of the house to the 25 minutes that you spend actually eating. I know this sounds terribly depressing, but believe it or not, you get used to it and will actually come to enjoy it. In a different way, of course.

Restaurant Dos and Don'ts: You Can Do It!

"Dear Miss Manners:
My husband has always let our son, who is now three, play
with various items on the table when we go out to eat.
These items include sugar packets, creamers, jelly packets,
and things of that nature. I think it's gross that they are
playing with things that other people will actually use
for their food and drink, but my husband thinks it's
no big deal because these items are wrapped."
Letter to syndicated newspaper column
Miss Manners © United Media (Miss Manners sides with
the writer of the letter in her response!)

There are some concrete guidelines that we follow to make sure that Willie and Daniel are in their best frame of mind for a restaurant experience. Making sure that they have had good naps that day, or are at least well-rested, is essential. I can trace many problems that we had in restaurants away from home to simple jet lag or travel fatigue. Also, we know that they should be hungry enough to look forward to the meal, but not "starving" to the point of being cranky and fussy. This sometimes requires a bit of schedule adjustment during the day, especially if our dinner plans are for later than they usually eat at home. If one of the boys is at all sick, plans are called off. After all, I don't particularly enjoy dining out when I'm not feeling well, so why should I expect them to? And during the day, we start talking to Willie, at least, about the plans to eat out that night, so that he, too, can start looking forward to it and incorporating the plans into his thinking.

If you're calling ahead to make a reservation, be sure to warn—I mean, inform—the restaurant that you will have young kids with you, and that you will need a high chair or booster seat at your table. If you have an infant who will stay in a carrier, I would tell them that, too, although you may find that the best spot for Baby is parked under the table or on a chair or bench next to you. Give the total number of people in your group, including all children, up front. I always say that we have a "party of four," and then mention that, by the way, two of them are children. There have been times that I've detected a subtle pause on the other end of the line, but, at least to date, no one has yet responded that kids are not welcome.

If you're at all anxious about this, by all means start with obviously family-friendly restaurants or, even better, small ethnic establishments. Talk to your child about the atmosphere and cuisine: "This is a Mexican restaurant; the food will be so good!" "At Chinese restaurants, sometimes people eat with chopsticks." If eating out is viewed as a Special Treat, that will go a long way toward getting full cooperation from your child. And if your schedule is at all adjustable, there is no question that it is usually easier for children to eat out on the early side. You may be the first reservation on the books at 5:30 or 6:00 p.m., but there is something to be said for getting in and out before the crowds arrive. Lunch is another good option to start with if you're really nervous; even the fanciest spots take on a more casual feel during the day. As far as restaurant layout goes, places with patios or outdoor tables are good choices. (Request this when you make a reservation if you know that outdoor seating is available.) It's probably totally psychological on my part, but I always feel less stared-at by other patrons if we're eating outdoors. I also like the feeling that we could drop cash on the table, gather up our stuff, and make a quick getaway if the situation truly disintegrates.

You should have a short list of items that you take with you every time you eat out; the items on the list will change with the age of your child. For a newborn or baby still in a carrier, you really won't need much at all, except maybe a bottle of pumped milk or formula if your meal will coincide with a regular feeding time. A few little toys, perhaps the kind that tie to the handle of the carrier, are a good idea, too, as is a pacifier if you have a baby who uses one. For an older baby or toddler who will be sitting at the table with you, the list might include a bib, a bottle or sippy cup, and perhaps a small plastic bag of Cheerios, to be pulled out in case of an emergency. Older kids shouldn't require any special gear. If you can get away with stuffing all of this into a large purse, do that, rather than carry it in an oversized diaper bag. Perhaps this is just me, but I always get more nervous in restaurants when I see parents toting in large bags of baby stuff or even baby gear like strollers and backpacks along with their child.

Two things you may have noticed missing from this list: a change of diapers, for young babies, and any sort of toy activities, for kids above the early toddler stage. Whether or not to take the diapers and accompanying items (wipes, creams, clean clothes, etc.) is of course your call, but I have found through experience that if you can get away without it for the brief time that you will probably be at the restaurant, it will greatly simplify your life. Many restaurant bathrooms are not equipped with changing tables or areas where you could put these things to use, so it's very likely that even if the need does arise, you will not be able to find a place to change Baby while you're at the restaurant anyway. (This is one reason why we have parking lots and cars with back seats.) It may make you feel more secure to have the diapers with you, but I can tell you from a lot of experience that the number of times that I have actually used them to change Willie or Daniel while we're at a restaurant is small, compared with the number of times that I've lugged the bag around and added one more item to keep track of. Again, your call, but in most cases, simplification wins every time.

Then there is the issue of toys at the table. Some restaurants will have them waiting at the front desk and will pull out coloring pages and such as soon as they see you in the doorway. On many occasions, I've been glad that I had the wayward crayon or two in my purse, to take up a little time before the food arrives. In general, I think that small toys like this—crayons, a little car, a small book—are a good idea to have on hand for very young children, in case they are needed. Don't pull them out if they are not, however; oftentimes, you may find that even little Toddler is perfectly happy watching the ceiling fan or the people around her. Distractions should be used only if necessary, lest they become an expectation at every outing and lose their "special" value.

There is one type of toy in particular, however, that I think should never be allowed at a restaurant or dinner table under any circumstances, and that is electronic gadgets such as DVD players or video games. In my interviews for this book, numerous chefs and restaurant managers told me that these hand-held electronics in the hands of dining kids are the bane of their existence, and that they'd actually rather have an unruly child in the dining room than one who is preoccupied by a light-up toy. Some have gone so far as to ban them from their restaurants completely, under the umbrella of "no cell phones." As Bob Carter, chef at the top-ranked Peninsula Grill in Charleston, South Carolina, told me: "We've grappled with this issue, because we've had some complaints about them. Electronic toys bother people at other tables because the pinging and the noise, and the lights that catch the corner of your eye are offensive to the dining experience." Carter, the father of two young sons himself, said that he completely understands that parents are simply trying to distract their tots with the use of items like DVDs, but adds that if parents are going to assume the responsibility of bringing their young children to nice restaurants, they need to be prepared to fully supervise and engage them, and not ignore them.

Chef Marc Murphy of New York's Landmarc restaurant spoke passionately about this issue when asked about his dining-out practices with his own five-year-old daughter and two-year-old son. "We'll usually bring some crayons if she wants to do some coloring, but we don't bring the television like a lot of other people do. It's crazy! What are you teaching? You can go and sit and not socialize. Once they're done with that, I guess they'll just move on to Blackberries in restaurants, so that'll be just great."

To practice and reinforce proper restaurant behavior, we have a game that we play with Willie, one we have oh-so-creatively dubbed "The Restaurant Game." Willie went through stages when he wanted to play this multiple times a day, and it can still bring a smile if Paul or I suggest it to him. In this game, Willie assumes the role of The Waiter and we of course are The Diners. He grabs a notepad and pen (or coloring book and crayon) and goes around to each person in the room, first listing the specials of the day. I know that he's been paying attention to some of our menu discussions when he comes up with some of his more visionary concepts, like smoked lettuce with blackened duck and cheese sauce, or shrimp with plums and applesauce, served with hot dogs and spaghetti on the side. We all go through the motions of placing orders for drinks, appetizers, salads, dinners ("and for your 'on-tray'?" Willie will ask) and desserts. He then becomes the chef who prepares the food, as well as the server, busboy, and cashier. Who knows where all of this is leading as far as any eventual professional interests go? For now, it's enough to say that it's a good way to familiarize him with the process and procedures of restaurant dining!

Please Be Seated

"Ian, do you want a cookie? Do you want some juice?
How about this cracker? Jason, get his train out
of the bag for him."
Obviously nervous mom, overheard while waiting for
a table at a busy upscale restaurant

When you bring a child with you to a restaurant, no matter what the age, you are bringing along another eater, another table conversationalist, another participant in the meal. I admit to many evenings out when I had wistful hopes of even ten minutes of interesting, adult table talk with Paul or whomever I was dining with, but ended up telling Willie another story about Thomas the Tank Engine or hearing his creative ramblings about what happened during his day. This is just another one of those things that you need to accept about life with young children! It is crucial to the success of your evening, as well as to the training process that you are working on with your children, to keep them engaged in the conversation. And that means talking *to* them and *with* them throughout the meal. Many chefs and restaurant managers told me that if they do have problems with children in their restaurant, it's often because of oblivious parents who act like they're out on a date or business dinner by themselves and just ignore the kids. I think that oftentimes, when parents say that their young children "can't sit still for long" at the dinner table, it simply is because they are not receiving enough attention.

The pacing and timing of your venture is very important. As soon as the host or hostess seats you and hands you menus, make a comment along the lines of "we'll be ready to order soon." This is a nice way of signaling to the staff that, yes, hello, "we know we have a child or children with us and we'll work with you to make this a good experience for everyone, including your other diners." Rearrange your table and the table settings to your own liking. (A smart waiter will help you with this, but if he or she just stands there cluelessly, plow ahead and do it yourself.) Position the infant carrier holder, high chair, or booster seat so that your child gets a view of something. Ceiling fans sometimes work well for babies; toddlers and preschoolers might like to watch the action in an open kitchen or be able to look out the window and see people go by. Move all of the sharp objects out of your child's reach, as well as anything that can turn into an inappropriate toy, like placemats, water glasses, packets of sweeteners, bud vases, and, in Willie's case, the salt and pepper shakers. Best to get all of this out of the way up front. If there is an extra napkin or two on the table, you might hold onto those, though. You never know when they might come in handy.

Learn to scan menus and make quick decisions about what to order. That way, as soon as the server brings you those first beverages or basket of bread, you're ready to go. If you let him or her get away by giving you "a few more minutes" to decide what you want, you waste precious time and run the risk that you won't see anyone who can take your order for some time. Better to get an order in quickly so that your food will be on the way, than to delay and have to entertain children while waiting. If you really want to study the menu, go to the restaurant's online Web site in the comfort of your own home or office before your visit and do your serious perusing there. Or ask for a menu before you are seated and take it outside to read. In the same manner, ask the server to bring you the check as soon as you receive your meals or dessert.

And no matter where you're dining, try to follow this rule: stay away from children's menus! A separate menu says to your toddler: because you are a child, we know what you will eat, and it's the same thing that every other child your age eats, over and over. Remember, *including* kids in the dining process is what is important to teaching restaurant manners and establishing harmony during the evening. *We all eat together* should be the mantra. For very young children, say, under the age of four, just let them share whatever foods and dishes that you order. As they get older, hungrier, and capable of eating more food, you can begin to order a separate dish for children. This can be something from the appetizer or salad menu if splurging for a full entrée would be an unnecessary waste.

It's also interesting to note that children's menus, for the most part, contain food items that are less healthful than the dishes offered on regular menus. This is similar to the comparison between child-oriented cereals and adult-oriented cereals, as we saw in Chapter 5. The consumer advocacy group Center for Science in the Public Interest investigated the kids' menus at 13 top national chain restaurants in 2008, and found that 93% of the featured items exceed 430 calories, one-third of the total amount that children ages four through eight should consume in one day. And guess what: 45% of the kids' fare items are also too high in saturated fat and 86% too high in sodium.[70] Too bad they didn't look at sugar content, too. More apparent evidence that not only are these Big Three–laden items bad on the nutritional front, but that overconsumption of one of them leads to overconsumption of another.

When placing your beverage order, ask the server to pour water or milk into your child's sippy cup. (You've remembered to stash one in your purse, along with a bib, right? No? Well, we've forgotten more times than I can count and have had to make do with a covered paper cup and straw, along with several oversized napkins, all provided by the restaurant.) If the minutes between placing the order and receiving the food are getting long or stressful, ask for more bread or other appropriate snacks (such as tortilla chips and guacamole in a Mexican restaurant) for your child to start on. Do not let them "fill up" on these, however. Rather than handing over an entire piece of bread, tear it off in bite-sized pieces and give these to your child one at a time. Giving them pieces of bread crust, rather than soft bread, will buy you a little extra time, too, as the crusts take a little longer to chew and swallow. Believe me, there will be times when every extra second counts!

For very young children (18–24 months or younger), bring along that small bag of Cheerios or other familiar snacks, but try to eliminate this practice as early as possible. Eating out should be a special occasion when everyone in the family tries something new or different, including children. Feeding them the same food that they would be eating at home defeats this message entirely, and does nothing to further the goal of broadening the palate and introducing new foods.

For kids who are old enough to understand the concept—say, three and up—bribing them for good behavior with a desired activity, like an extra bedtime story, can be a helpful tactic. A favorite dessert could be delivered at the restaurant immediately following the meal ("I hear they have a wonderful apple tart; shall we try some after dinner?"), or something like a scoop of ice cream once you get home. Stick to your guns on this one, though: if you tell them that they have to act in a certain way to get the goodies, then any infraction is grounds for a "sorry, not this time."

One other important point, for those of you who love your cocktail or glass of pinot noir with dinner as much as I do: watch how much you drink at dinner. A glass of restaurant-pour wine in the large glasses that they typically use may be more than a single serving and contain more wine (alcohol) than you realize. It's nice to get a relaxed effect, but not too relaxed! The cute toddler in the high chair or preschooler in a booster seat still needs your close attention.

I've been told by several restaurant managers that this is particularly a problem with diners who come in groups: everyone is there to have a good time together (which the restaurant wants); all of the adults start drinking together (which the restaurant also wants), and all of a sudden, no one is paying any attention to the kids in the group (which the restaurant hates). The children get bored or whiny and start sliding out of their seats, tossing napkins, or, as a maitre d' at one Four Seasons Hotel remembers, "sitting down on the floor, right in the middle of the dining room, and refusing to move."

Tactful waiters will come up with lines for the parents, such as "we're concerned about your child's safety; we don't want someone to trip over her." They will pull out coloring books and crayons or little hand toys and generally do anything possible to keep *your child* from causing a scene, including, at the top establishments, offering the services of an employee to take the child for a walk. But what they really want to say is, "Parents, please deal with your kids!"

With all of this in mind, I hope that it doesn't sound too contradictory to say that there is also a lot of value in simply relaxing when you're out to dinner with your kids. If you're worked up over their behavior, chances are that some of that nervousness will transfer to the kids, resulting in even more problems. Remember that as long as your children are even reasonably well-behaved, most people around you, even at the nicest of restaurants, will not be annoyed by the fact that they are there. And if you can pull off a behavior-perfect evening, people will marvel at your parenting skills. The best advice I can give you to help you achieve that is to just keep moving through your meal in a steady, comfortable pace, keeping a close eye on the situation so that you're ready to bolt quickly if things really fall apart. Smile a lot.

And if a meltdown does occur, don't hang your head in shame; I can almost guarantee you that the restaurant staff has seen worse and that, as long as you deal properly with the situation, most of the other diners feel empathy toward you, rather than anger or resentment. Know when it's time to go, pay your bill quickly, and move on. Don't spend a lot of time apologizing or even attempting to clean up if your toddler has made a mess of the floor or table. I've been told by many restaurateurs that it's helpful to the staff if you can pick up some of the big pieces of food that may have fallen to the floor, or put a napkin over a water spill, but let them take care of the rest. The last thing they need is you crawling around under the table on all fours, trying to scoop up every far-flung grain of rice. As chef Marc Murphy of Restaurant Landmarc said, many waiters actually love to get tables with kids, as the parents often feel guilty about the extra work and mess that they are causing, and leave tips to reflect that!

And above all, take heart in knowing that this time, too, shall pass. If you start these restaurant experiences early enough, and make them a regular part of your kids' lives as they are growing up, it will amaze you how quickly they will become accustomed to the whole process. One night you may be out with them and suddenly realize that, wait a minute, yes, we can stay around for dessert, or that it doesn't matter that your server messed up the check and it's going to take an extra 20 minutes to straighten it out. The kids are *behaving* and everyone is really having fun. They are dining in a restaurant, and they know what's expected of them.

When Willie was about 27 months old, we visited Hawaii for the first time. While on the beautiful island of Maui, we discovered the little gem Chez Paul, a distinctly French restaurant with a bit of Hawaiian flair. On our last night on the island, we booked a table. It was a Saturday night, traditionally the busiest night in the restaurant world, and we could only get an 8:00 p.m. reservation. Our waitress was most gracious, mentioning that she, too, had a child about the same age and how nice it was to see one so young being schooled in the art of dining.

As we finished our wonderful dinner and were preparing to leave, a couple seated nearby stopped by our table. The woman wanted us to know that when she saw us come in, she was immediately filled with dread that "a child" was seated so close to their table, during a dinner that was held to celebrate an important and happy occasion. She said that she even briefly considered complaining to the management. "Never again will I prejudge a young child in a restaurant," she said. "It's nice to see that it can be done."

Super Success Stories

"Daddy, this is the best veal carpaccio and arugula I've ever had!"
Comment overheard in a swanky Vail, Colorado, restaurant,
from a table where a five-kid family dined together

Every now and then, you hear stories about young kids who will truly eat anything. These are the ones who seemingly can be taken to any restaurant in the world, to any person's house, anywhere, and they not only will happily eat whatever is presented to them but will do so with gusto. Some of them may grow up to be the tweens who are flocking to cooking schools and camps and are bona fide foodies by the age of ten or twelve. Kitchen retailer Williams-Sonoma latched onto this bunch and started a line of cooking tools and equipment for children, as well as cooking classes. "Kids are really interested in food," said Williams-Sonoma spokesperson Hilleary Kehrli. A generation that has grown up with The Food Network and celebrity chefs, she adds, "is seeing it all on TV, and that continues the tradition of kids learning to cook from their parents and grandparents."[71]

In research for this book, I ran into quite a few of these kids. Do the parents have any secrets on how to pull this off, I wondered, anything that they could share with those of us whose children have, shall we say, different abilities?

It's interesting to note that not all of these super-success-story kids were born with the proverbial silver spoon in their mouths. While some of them did come from families who have the means to eat out often, shop at the designer-name grocery stores, and take trips to exotic locations, that was not true in all cases. In fact, I found many more instances where the upper-crust kids were the most white-bread in their approach to food. Perhaps as an extension of being catered to in other ways, a lot of these kids are also allowed to make too many food choices on their own.

One common theme in many of these superstar eaters: some strong connection to another country or another culture, outside of the United States. Go figure.

My friend Niccole, married to a Bolivian, has a five-year-old son who is definitely top-eater caliber. We're talking about a kid who snacks on sardines with onions and Roquefort, insists on anchovies across a pizza and the sweetbread appetizer at a restaurant, and vigorously consumes all kinds of South American dishes such as ranga (described to me as cow stomach stewed in tomato sauce), anticuchos (grilled heart of beef), and marrowbones. His American side also likes Oreos, hot dogs, and "this weird casserole that his grandmother makes that features Velveeta cheese and cream of mushroom soup." Niccole is the first to tell you that she and her husband brought their son up in this style of eating and have worked from early on to teach him to love and to respect food.

"We eat everything, sautéed and deep-fried, as well as broiled or steamed," Niccole says. "I use full fat everything, never anything 'low fat' or 'artificially sweetened.' Nothing gets 'dumbed down' for him. If a recipe calls for chili or wine or 18 cloves of garlic, it goes in and he eats the same thing that we do. But I do keep portion sizes small, more like we eat in South America, rather than the typical American Cheesecake Factory size."

I asked Niccole what she remembers about her son's eating as a toddler, and whether or not she thought her early feeding routine had anything to do with his broad palate now. It turns out that she did make all of his baby food from the first days, boiling and pureeing vegetables to start, and quickly adding textures and whole foods. Niccole insists that this was no major effort, and the results obviously made it worthwhile. "I remember seeing a jar of pureed peas for babies, and it was gray. No wonder babies don't like vegetables," she added. "If I had to choose between applesauce and gray peas, I'd probably go with the fruit every time too."

Matthew Forney is a distinguished newspaper journalist who lives with his Italian-born wife and two young children in Beijing. He is also working on a book about his family's life in China. As you might imagine, that life has included an introduction to food items that would be considered a bit bizarre here in the United States. When you talk about kids who will eat anything, these two appear to be at the top of the list.

Scorpions! Goat testicles! Sichuanese snails and Tibetan yak jerky! "This is what eating is like in my household," Forney writes in a *New York Times* column. "My children eat anything. Think of a child staging a sit-in at his suburban dinner table because there's a fleck of dried parsley on his breaded fish finger, and you have imagined everything my children are not."[72]

I'll say. Forney readily admits in his piece that he's not sure if he and his wife deserve credit for rearing such adventurous eaters.

They point out that in countries like China, where poverty has been, and sometimes continues to be, a common issue, people "learn to eat what's available or they starve. Fussiness never enters the picture." So children absorb an entirely different attitude about food. He also adds that, at their Chinese nursery school, his kids were fed—and expected to eat—a standard Chinese meal that included such items as pickled turnips, flakes of dough sticks, green or red beans, sesame paste, and something called hot prickly mustard tubers. And they did.

"Have I got some kids for you," the sommelier at a top Charleston, South Carolina, restaurant told me by way of introduction to the children of a local businessman. "One of them was here last night with his dad, sitting perfectly through a long meal and trying a little bit of everything we brought out. He loves our snails and mussel soup. Last night, he let the chef know that he couldn't taste the oysters in his oysters casino because there was a tad too much bacon. The chef tasted the dish, agreed, and sent out another plate." This child is five years old.

This man says that all four of his children, ages six, five, three, and one, are superstar eaters, thanks to the efforts that he and his wife have made to teach them about good food. "I make an effort to take the kids out individually for some one-on-one time at restaurants," he said. "This exposes them to high-end dining and, with concentrated attention, they have learned how to eat and how to behave." One of his daughters spent her sixth birthday eating at the Senate Dining Room in Washington, D.C., and later at Citronelle, one of the city's finest. They all loved the sushi at Masa in New York (where dinner averages about $400 a person) but were less than impressed with the sandwiches and brownie sundaes at touristy Rockefeller Center. The kids have traveled through Europe, eating at some of the best restaurants in Paris and Rome. They've learned to assess restaurants not only for the quality of food, but for the level of service and the atmosphere.

His advice for other parents who want to instill this level of appreciation for food at such a young age? "Take them out a lot; it's all about practice. Go early, before the serious crowds. Look at the menus on Web sites ahead of time, and tell them what they may be eating. Dress them up and make it a special event, so that their behavior will rise to the occasion. Let them know that experiences like this are a privilege, earned by their good behavior. They are expected to be neat and polite and thankful to the staff.

"Eat with them at home and talk to them about what they are eating. We also have a 'you have to try it' rule when it comes to new foods. You can leave it on your plate if it's something you don't like, but you do have to try."

This foodie-dad adds that all of this is well worth it in the end, because it makes dining out so much more fun for the adults involved. "You get to see things through their eyes," he says. "What could be better than sharing experiences like this with family?"

What I've Learned

— It's really important, for both you and your kids, that you take them out to eat at restaurants, starting early in their lives, and going often. Pulling this off smoothly is a skill. As with learning any new skill, you may feel nervous at first but will gain confidence with practice and experience. One failure is not the end of the road.

— If you're worried about what other diners may think of you or your kids, keep in mind that you are judged harshly only if you don't deal appropriately with behavior problems. Handle situations as they arise, and people will forgive just about anything.

— Most important in a restaurant with children is teaching them the concept of *dining together*. Parking the kids at the table with a DVD or other all-encompassing electronic toy so that the adults can have their own time does nothing to further this.

— No matter where you choose to eat, you can do better than the children's menu. Best for your kids not even to know that these exist. Besides being traps of dishes that contain too much fat, sodium, and sugar, these items do not have enough interest or flavor variation to give your kids any kind of real experience with food.

— The kids you know who are truly superstar eaters, or can be taken to any type of restaurant and counted on to behave beautifully, have parents who have worked at this. It did not "just happen," and the parents did not "just get lucky," no matter what they say!

CHAPTER 10

⌘

Cheers!

Despite your best efforts to teach your child about the enjoyment of food, and to school their little palates so they will enjoy eating a broader spectrum, there are times that it Just Won't Work. Maybe it's when you discover that a babysitter has been treating your child to candy and snacks more frequently than you'd like, as I once did, or when they return from a grandparent's house with a newfound love of Oreos. No matter how carefully you try to supervise the diet, there will be occasions when it's out of your control and influence. And it's those times that you have to relax, trust what you're doing at home, and just give in a bit.

Although some statements in this book may seem a little contradictory to this point, I have never worried too much about foods that William or Daniel eat when they are not with me, simply because I know how they both eat at home. And as long as they are learning the proper lessons about food choice here, a few less-than-perfect snack foods or ill-timed sweets will not undo everything that I am trying to accomplish. In fact, there is a lot to be said for not making any foods the "forbidden treats," which, in the end, may only make them more appealing. When Willie spots the Golden Arches and says "I like those hamburgers," or references the "yummy Jell-O and candy" he ate in playgroup, I gloss right over it and move on to the next subject.

The whole key is to set firm standards, adhere to them for the long term as much as possible, but always remember that food, dining, and eating are supposed to be Fun. Anguishing over diets is not effective for anyone and sends young children the message that food is something to be scrutinized, rather than enjoyed.

Willie himself reminded Paul and me of this during one of our dinners out, this time at a wonderful local seafood restaurant in Florida. Paul was there on a business trip and Willie and I had decided to tag along, as it was the middle of February and we were tired of the cold Washington winter. We had all enjoyed the trip together, eating out at many wonderful Miami restaurants. This was, in fact, the trip on which we discovered that our boy liked to eat octopus.

At the end of the week, some of Paul's business acquaintances invited us all to dinner. Even though the trip and restaurant ventures had been successful to that point, dining out with people we didn't know well was something that still made me a little nervous. When Paul told me that they had chosen a restaurant 40 miles away in Fort Lauderdale, and that we had a dinner reservation for 9:00 p.m., I nearly panicked, pleading, "Didn't you tell them you're bringing a two-year-old?" (The only thing that made this slightly easier for me was the fact that Paul was the client and that these particular people really wanted to sign a business deal with him. I figured that they would put up with just about anything to get that contract.)

We arrived at the restaurant right on time, only to be told that our table wouldn't be ready for another 30 minutes. We had no choice but to move to the crowded bar area, where basketball-loving fans were hooting and hollering through a close NBA game. We moved with little Willie to a side table, where he, fortunately, sat back and took in the action.

It seemed forever until we were finally seated, but before long, we were enjoying appetizers and a beautiful wine. Willie, seated beside me in his high chair, had his sippy cup filled with water and a slice of lemon, "for flavor," as he told the waiter. Just as we were preparing to enjoy the wine, Willie raised his sippy cup and said "Cheers, Daddy!" He then leaned over to touch the glass of each person at the table, giggling "Cheers" throughout each "toast."

Yes, "Cheers." It was then that I knew that we were definitely off to a good start with this little boy.

Can You Take This Too Far?

"My husband and I are control freaks about the foods that our son eats. He's never had nonorganic vegetables, processed sugar, or anything from a can. The one problem that we have with him now that he's three is that he has discovered store-bought mayonnaise. He wants it on everything. He started crying the other day in the grocery store, begging me to buy a jar."
Jennifer, mother of a three-and-a-half year-old

Somewhere in your group of parent-friends, you may run into the Mom or Dad who sees her- or himself as the Captain of the Food Police. These people subscribe to the theory that a child's diet requires strict management, as opposed to guidance. For health reasons, for food safety reasons, perhaps for religious reasons or other factors known only unto them, there are parents who very strictly monitor and control exactly what their children eat. Every food is scrutinized and deemed either acceptable or no-go; very few, if any, exceptions are allowed. You may not encounter many of these types, but the ones whom you do will be adamant in their convictions.

Is this a smart strategy? Does strict denial of certain foods now lead to food abstinence later in life? What other behaviors are affected?

"My daughter has been in daycare/preschool since she was four months old, and she was only allowed to eat home-cooked food at school," one mother of a four-year-old told me. "This is part of a larger situation in which she was not exposed to conventional foods until recently. My husband was adamant that she have the best possible nutrition, even if he had to make it from scratch—fresh and organic—every morning. Occasionally, she was allowed to eat in restaurants and at other people's homes, but was not allowed to eat things like hamburgers and hot dogs, chicken nuggets, fish sticks, fast foods, and other animal products. We don't use condiments at home because we don't believe in masking the real flavor of food with enhancements.

"For a long time, I was concerned that all of this was starting to affect her psychologically. She didn't want to eat her home-cooked lunch at school, or ate very little of it. She would be very hungry for the rest of the afternoon or even steal other kids' food! After a while, she was growing despondent. She was too hungry to sleep during naptime, and she saw all the other kids eating the same lunch, served in the same kinds of plates, while her food was different-looking and -tasting and served in a different container. We tried to mitigate this issue by reviewing the school's menu each day and preparing a lunch that was similar—like packing a chicken-like noodle soup when the school was serving chicken noodle soup. And we talked to the teachers to make sure that her food was served in paper plates just like the others'. We did this for a whole year. She wasn't malnourished, because she was eating very well at home, but we could see that it was affecting her psyche and her relationships with schoolmates.

"My husband finally cracked. We were juggling a more complex morning routine of his new job, plus preparing all the food for my daughter and our newborn. I broached the subject again because I was concerned and he finally relented, on one condition. He sat my daughter down and talked to her about it, saying he was allowing her now to eat school food on the condition that she still drink her veggie-fruit morning shake and eat an organic, freshly cooked dinner. It was like a dam burst—she was a different child at school. She became more confident and outgoing, she pays greater attention in class, and she actually takes naps. And as she started eating conventional foods, she discovered ketchup and is now obsessed about putting it on just about anything she eats.

"For us, it was a big lesson. After all, kids are very social creatures and even at an early age they can be conscious of their social environment."

This story may be out of the ordinary in its intensity, but the message is supported by research on the effects of out-and-out "food denial." One potentially negative outcome: overindulgence in unhealthful foods, when not even hungry.

Baylor University researcher Jennifer Fisher of the Children's Nutrition Research Center observed the eating habits of nearly 200 five-year-old girls over a two-year period to see what and how much of several tempting snack foods they would consume right after eating a full meal and were no longer hungry. Fisher also looked at parental restriction of the snack foods used in the study and even assessed the children's perception of that parental restriction.

No surprise initially; Fisher found that, despite their reported lack of hunger, few of the girls could resist the temptation to nibble on at least some of the ten snack foods offered to them. But what was interesting was that she found that some of the girls did just that—nibble—while others consistently consumed a lot of the foods even when they weren't hungry.

The difference? The girls whose parents most tightly controlled their overall diets at the age of five ate significantly more snack calories when out of their parents' view than did those with less controlling parents. And of course, those who ate the most snacks when not hungry were more than four times as likely to be overweight at both five and seven years of age.[73]

And at Penn State, researchers also found that forbidden foods were perceived by young children to be more desirable. Kids were given access to apple or peach cookie bars, things that they had rated as "just OK" in an earlier taste test. Some of the bars were served on plates, while others were placed in clear cookie jars in the middle of the table. The children were told that after ten minutes, they could snack on cookies from the jar. Restricting those cookies really had a profound effect; consumption of the cookies in the jars was more than triple that of those on the plates.[74]

So it seems that the answer to the original question is yes, you can take all of this too far. It's definitely possible to put too much emphasis on foods chosen, rather than foods enjoyed. Hearing "No, you can't eat that" too often may bring the response, "Oh, yes I can, and I will," as your child grows into a decision maker in his own right. After all, kids don't like to be told what to do any more than the rest of us.

Maybe, then, the answer to the parental quandary of exactly how much control to exert over the diet is found somewhere in the middle of the spectrum. Our job as parents is to teach, to lead, and to expose. Part of a child's learning in food education involves experimentation, which may lead to failure, at least in the eyes of the teacher. A sudden love of a "bad food," even one that turns into a long-term food jag, may be viewed as just that—a failure. But if Mom and Dad maintain their lessons as the preferred standards, with consistency, with love, and with a dash of humor when appropriate, eventually, the student will return to those teachings.

Where Does It All Lead?

"My boys have grown up eating whatever I prepared from scratch, even as infants. No jarred baby food for them. We've cooked, grocery shopped, and eaten together since they were very young. Now they're young men and there is still nothing we would rather do than cook or dine together. It's part of the way we stay connected."
Bonnie, food columnist, mother of 25-year-old and 28-year-old sons

As with most aspects of childrearing, there can be a certain amount of tedium involved in all of this.

Feeding kids day in and day out is never easy, but if you take on the additional task of trying to add some quality, some flavor, some nutritional and taste value, some real meaning to what they consume—well, if you're like me, there will be many times that you yourself will have had enough. There have been plenty of occasions when I've questioned the point of stepping out on this limb, wondered if it's worth the hassle, and been very tempted to relent more than I should. I mean, so many other kids and their parents don't seem to give a whit about what they eat, and they seem fine. Do we really need to add a layer of complication?

And then I meet people like Di-Anna Arias of San Antonio, a catering sales director at the acclaimed Don Strange of Texas and a co-owner of Earl Able's Restaurant, a city landmark for more than 60 years. When Di-Anna and her husband returned home from a recent trip to New York, their son Jordan eagerly awaited his gift from the Big Apple. A Knicks jersey? A new CD? Nope, for this 16-year-old, it was a bottle of first-press olive oil and a balsamic vinegar that they found at a small grocery store. "And his eyes just lit up at the sight of it," his mother recounts. "He was immediately off to Central Market to buy some bread to try it.

"This is not a complication," Di-Anna corrected me. "It's a personal value that we want to instill in him. And it's a value that represents so many other things, namely a healthy body and a curious mind. What better way to teach kids about their world and the people in it than to teach them about the food that we all eat?

"So we brought Jordan up to love food," she said. "It started years ago, with me making his own baby food. Jordan never ate commercial baby food. I just could not bring myself to open up a jar of food that had been sitting on a grocery store shelf since who knows when and one that contained preservatives."

Uh-huh.

"I remember when he was about three, we went to his cousins' house and the kids had canned ravioli for lunch," she continued. "My sister-in-law still teases him about his comment: 'Aunt Cindy, this doesn't taste right!' It wasn't said in a mean or snotty way, it was just an astute observation.

"We also started taking him to restaurants at a very young age. When he was five years old, he knew how to order his steak—the soft one, tenderloin—and when he would order a latté at the end of the meal, the waitress would just look at us, sometimes with disagreement, but I figured that since my great-grandparents began drinking coffee at three or four years of age and lived into their late 90s, what do I have to worry about? To this day, coffee is one of his favorite things in the world.

"And then there was his school lunch. He took his lunch every day because he could not stand the selection in the cafeteria. Usually his lunches included a great sandwich of turkey, pesto sauce, cheese and greens, and sometimes a slice of cake from home or a wedge of Brie with crackers. His friends would wonder what was for lunch each day. Many times he took extra to share."

I asked Di-Anna what benefits she and her husband are now reaping, and how their perseverance through the years paid off. Give us parents of younger kids some encouragement, I said. Are we on the right track?

"Eating together is something that you should look forward to, no matter if it is a pizza and salad or you bring out the good china, it is a meal together," she said. "We never did the 'eating in the car' thing, and still don't. If our son has a commitment around dinner time, dinner is planned a little earlier or later. Remember that you have control of their time when they are young. You can teach them so many basic manners—how to hold a knife and fork, how to order in a restaurant, how to excuse yourself from the table, thanking the server.

"And all these years later," she continued, "we have a handsome, popular teenage son who has a knowledge and love and appreciation for food, far beyond what I see in most of his friends," she said. "It's something that will serve him well for the rest of his life, both from a health and nutrition point of view, and an intellectual perspective, as I've seen how it broadens his mind and encourages creativity.

"It's something we will always share together as a family."

Let It Be

"With my daughter, I spent a lot of time and energy worrying about what she ate. Everything had to be nutritious, or at least all-natural, organic, or healthful in some way. When the second child came along, I threw in the towel. I didn't have the time or energy to preach about it any more and in the end, I'm not sure it matters anyway. My oldest now loves junk food and the younger one is the budding chef, obsessed with what he calls 'quality cuisine.' So there you go."
Debbie, mother of two young adults

This book would not be complete without a summary of the "how-to-get-kids-to-eat" theory espoused by numerous experts consulted for this text, from the writings of Clara Davis to Benjamin Spock, to prominent food journalists, such as Raymond Solokov and David Kamp, to chefs, nutrition experts, and researchers, as well as many average American moms and dads. And that is the idea that we, as parents, should simply relax about this whole issue, stop making such a big deal over what our children do or do not eat, and trust that they will eventually develop mature and even enlightened palates, suitable for the adult world.

The sum of much of this advice is simple: wait it out, with the understanding that all children will be forced to adapt to a grown-up world of food in time. "Just give them whatever they want for a while," says acclaimed food writer Raymond Sokolov, currently of the *Wall Street Journal*'s "Eating Out" column and author of numerous cookbooks and food histories. "Young children will give up their transitory dietary phobias when they go to school, as no one else will tolerate them like they do at home."

My friend Susan, a Washington, D.C. chef and mother of two sons, agrees, adding, "I was a picky eater as a child, and now I'm a chef. Just present foods and don't make a big deal out of what they eat and what they don't. The point is to get to adulthood exposed to a lot of foods. Everyone will have likes and dislikes along the way." The prolific food journalist David Kamp, a New Yorker who has some of the best restaurants in the world at his feet, remembers that as a child he didn't like steak or raw tomatoes. His wife, too, was an extremely picky eater in her youth. Yet as adults they are both food-lovers. And now they have a son who won't eat pasta. They don't focus so much on their children's culinary likes and dislikes because, as Kamp says, "I've seen in my own life how the evolution to an appreciation of food works."

This is, in some ways, the easiest solution of all, as it requires only that we stop the excessive fretting. And to this excellent piece of advice, I would add two small caveats: don't worry, but don't ignore the issue, and don't succumb, either.

Don't give up by deciding that the palate development of your kids is out of your control, or not important enough to spend time on. Don't give up the practice of taking them to nice restaurants just because you experience a one-time disaster that makes you feel like you can never show your face on that street again. Don't stop cooking with your kids, or taking them grocery-shopping with you or to a farmer's market, simply because, as they get older, other activities will seem to take on more importance. What they eat as children, what they come to learn and think about food, will in many ways be with them for the rest of their lives.

And, please, to the best of your ability, don't succumb to the power of the rampant forces that you will find to be working against you in all of this. As your child hits the preschool years, especially, it may seem as though you are the only person in the world who cares whether children consume chicken Cordon Bleu or fried chicken nuggets, real apples or apple candies, milk or Mountain Dew. I have been in groups of kids where virtually none of them eat with their family or have any concept that vegetables actually grow in the ground. It's amazing how many will tell you that a restaurant is a place "where you go to a counter or a window to pick up food," and that their parents regularly have them eat in the car.

Just remember this: if you want your child to love food and to enjoy the riches that it can bring to her life, you have to tell her about it. You have to show her the way, teach her to discern the good from the bad, the ripe from the not-yet-ready, the knock-off from the real thing. Kids are a complete blank slate in this regard. Your years of influence over their thoughts and behavior may be few, but they are very powerful. Take advantage of that, and make your home, at least, the one place that your children will come to count on for guidance in eating the "best" foods. As so many chefs and others told me, it is the messages that kids receive from their parents, from the home, that will eventually win out. The culture may be working against you, but the great consensus that

I heard was that if children are simply exposed to good food at home, on a consistent basis and from a young age, they will grow to be able to make their own proper food choices.

What else have I learned through this project? When I started this book, I had an adorable two-year-old who ate octopus as readily as most toddlers eat yogurt or fruit. He's since grown into an energetic five-year-old who displays a broad palate and an adventurous attitude toward food, the occasional independence-laced rebellion notwithstanding. I will say that, at this point, he is a better eater than just about any other child his age whom I know, at least most of the time. Ask him what he wants for dinner tonight, and he's as likely as any kid to say "pizza." But if I push him a bit—"come on, Willie, what about Greek food, or maybe this new casserole recipe?"—he can be convinced.

I've also added to the mix a new two-year-old, who, to date, will eventually eat anything put before him, although with a little more trepidation and refusal at times than First Son typically showed. Just the other day, though, the boys were in our backyard looking at the tomato plants, and I heard Willie say to Daniel: "You can only pick the red ones. The green ones aren't ripe yet." I savored that as one of those little victories I'm always looking for.

How will it all turn out? Who knows—ask me in ten or twenty years and maybe I can give a good answer. I just hope that I can say then that they are both still eating octopus, and anything else new that is put before them, with the curiosity and the enthusiasm of a two-year-old.

⌘

Notes and References

1 Neerguard, L. "Bad News for American Kids: Rickets on the Rise." Associated Press, November 26, 2007.

2 Gerber Feeding Infants and Toddlers Study (FITS). March–July 2002. Published in *Journal of the American Dietetic Association*, 2004; 104: 31–37.

3 "Tooth Decay among Preschool Children on the Rise," National Center for Health Statistics, Centers for Disease Control and Prevention, April 2007.

4 Davis, C. M. "Results of the Self-Selection of Diets by Young Children." *Canadian Medical Association Journal*, 1939; 41:257–261.

5 Davis, C. M. "Self Selection of Diet by Newly Weaned Infants: An Experimental Study." *American Journal of Diseases of Children*, 1928; 36(4):651–679.

6 Harrison, K. "Nutritional Content of Foods Advertised During the Television Programs Children Watch Most." *American Journal of Public Health*, September 2005.

311

7 Kunkel, D. "Report of the APA Task Force on Advertising and Children." Report to the American Psychological Association, February 2004.

8 Nestle, M. "Food Marketing and Childhood Obesity." *New England Journal of Medicine*, June 2006; 354:2527–2529.

9 Koivisto, U. K., and Sjoden, P. O. "Reasons for Rejection of Food Items in Swedish Families with Children Aged 2–17." *Appetite*, 1996; 26:89–104.

10 Skinner, J., et al. "Toddlers' Food Preferences: Concordance with Family Members' Preferences." *Journal of Nutrition Education*, 1998; 30:17–22.

11 Carruth, B. R., and Skinner, J. "Revisiting the Picky Eater Phenomenon: Neophobic Behaviors of Young Children." *Journal of the American College of Nutrition*, 2000; 19:771–780.

12 Mennella, J. A., et al. "Garlic Ingestion by Pregnant Women Alters the Odor of Amniotic Fluid." *Chemical Senses*, 1995; 20:207–209.

13 Hepper, P. G. "Human Fetal Olfactory Learning." *International Journal of Prenatal and Perinatal Psychology and Medicine*, 1995; 7:147–151.

14 Schaal, B., et al. "Olfactory Function in the Human Fetus: Evidence from Selective Neonatal Responsiveness to the Odor of Amniotic Fluid." *Behavioral Neurosciences*, 1998; 112(6):1438–1439.

15 Schaal, B., et al. "Human Foetuses Learn Odours from Their Pregnant Mother's Diet." *Chemical Senses*, 2000; 25:729–737.

16 Mennella, J. A., et al. "Prenatal and Postnatal Flavor Learning by Human Infants." *Pediatrics*, 2001; 107(6):E88.

17 Gerrish, C. J., and Mennella, J. A. "Flavor Variety Enhances Food Acceptance in Formula-Fed Infants." *American Journal of Clinical Nutrition*, 2001; 73(6):1080–1085.

18 Harris, G. "More Mothers Breast-Feed, in First Months at Least." *New York Times*, May 1, 2008.

19 Baumslag, N., and Michels, D. L. *Milk, Money and Madness: The Culture and Politics of Breastfeeding.* Bergin & Garvey Trade, 1995.

20 Ibid.

21 Skinner, J. D., et al. "Do Food-Related Experiences in the First 2 Years of Life Predict Dietary Variety in School-Aged Children?" *Journal of Nutrition Education and Behavior*, 2002; 34:310–315.

22 Forestall, C. A., and Mennella, J. A. "Early Determinants of Fruit and Vegetable Acceptance." *Pediatrics,* 2007; 120(6):1247–1254.

23 Ibid.

24 Mennella, J. A., et al. "Vegetable Acceptance by Infants: Effects of Formula Flavors." *Early Human Development,* 2006; 82(7):463–468.

25 Mennella, J. A., and Beauchamp, G. K. "Flavor Experiences During Formula Feeding Are Related to Preferences During Childhood." *Early Human Development,* 2002, 68(2):71–82.

26 Cashdan, E. "A Sensitive Period for Learning about Food." *Human Nature,* 1994; 5(3):279–291.

27 Birch, L. L., et al. "Children's Eating: The Development of Food-Acceptance Patterns." *Young Children,* 1995; 50(2):71–78.

28 Ibid.

29 Ibid.

30 Skinner, J., et al. "Toddlers' Food Preferences: Concordance with Family Members' Preferences." *Journal of Nutrition Education,* 1998; 30:17–22.

31 Rozin, P. "The Nature of Preference for Peppers." *Behav Emo,* 1980; 4:77–101.

32 Stallone, D. D., and Jacobson, M. F. "Cheating Babies: Nutritional Quality and Cost of Commercial Baby Food." Center for Science in the Public Interest Report.

33 Keskitalo, K., et al. "Sweet Taste Preferences are Partly Genetically Determined: Identification of a Trait Locus on Chromosome 16." *American Journal of Clinical Nutrition,* 2007; 86(1):55–63.

34 Cloud, J. "Eating Better Than Organic." *Time Magazine,* March 2, 2007.

35 Paddock, C. "Organic Food Is More Nutritious, Say EU Researchers." *Medical News Today,* October 29, 2007.

36 Theuer, R. C. "Do Organic Fruits and Vegetables Taste Better Than Conventional Produce?" Organic Center Study, December 2006.

37 Skinner, J. D., et al. "Do Food-Related Experiences in the First Two Years of Life Predict Dietary Variety in School-Aged Children?" *Journal of Nutrition Education and Behavior,* 2002; 34(6):310–315.

38 Cashdan, E. "A Sensitive Period for Learning about Food." *Human Nature,* 1994; 5(3):279–291.

39 Birch, L. L., et. al. "Children's Eating: The Development of Food-Acceptance Patterns." *Young Children,* 1995; 50(2):71–78.

40 Skinner, J., et al. "Toddlers' Food Preferences: Concordance with Family Members' Preferences." *Journal of Nutrition Education,* 1998; 30:17–22.

41 Carruth, B. R., and Skinner, J. "Revisiting the Picky Eater Phenomenon: Neophobic Behaviors of Young Children." *Journal of the American College of Nutrition,* 2000; 19:771–780.

42 "Managing Early Childhood Obesity in the Primary Care Setting." *Pediatric Nursing,* 2002; 28(6):599–610.

43 Birch, L. L., et al. "Children's Eating: The Development of Food-Acceptance Patterns." *Young Children,* 1995; 50(2):71–78.

44 Song, W. O., et al. "Ready-to-Eat Breakfast Cereal Consumption Enhances Milk and Calcium Intake in the U.S. Population." *Journal of the American Dietetic Association,* 2006; 106(11):1783–1789.

45 Falci, L. "Mass of US Breakfast Cereal Consumption." *Physics Factbook,* 2006.

46 Beauchamp, G. "Reduced-Sodium Strategy." Presentation to preparedfoods.com, May 2008.

47 *Retailer Daily,* May 6, 2006.

48 American Academy of Pediatrics, Committee on Nutrition. "The Use and Misuse of Fruit Juice in Pediatrics." *Pediatrics,* 2001; 107(5): 1210–1213.

49 Wang, Y. C., et al. "Increasing Caloric Contribution from Sugar-Sweetened Beverages and 100% Fruit Juices among U.S. Children and Adolescents, 1998–2004." *Pediatrics,* 2008; 121(6):1604–1614.

50 Dennison, B. A. "Excess Fruit Juice Consumption by Preschool-Age Children Is Associated with Short Stature and Obesity." *Pediatrics,* 1997; 99(1):15–22.

51 *USDA Continuing Survey of Food Intakes by Individuals, 1994–1996.* 1998.

52 From testimony to Federal Drug Administration, November 29, 2007, by American Medical Association Vice President for Science, Quality and Public Health Stephen Havas, MD, MPH, MS.

53 Wooten, M. G. "Pestering Parents: How Food Companies Market Obesity to Children." *Center for Science in the Public Interest Reports,* November 2003.

54 Telephone poll conducted by Widmeyer Commications for the Center for a New American Dream. May 2002. 750 American youth ages 12–17 participated. Margin of error ±3.5%.

55 Marr, K. "Children Targets of $1.6 Billion in Food Ads: FTC Discloses 2006 Spending in First-Ever Report." *Washington Post,* July 30, 2008. D-1.

56 Nestle, M. "Food Marketing and Childhood Obesity." *New England Journal of Medicine,* June 2006; 354:2527–2529.

57 Robinson, T. N., et al. "Effects of Fast Food Branding on Young Children's Taste Preferences." *Archives of Pediatrics & Adolescent Medicine,* August 2007; 161(8):792–797.

58 *USDA Continuing Survey of Food Intakes by Individuals, 1994–1996.* 1998.

59 Wang, Y. C., et al. "Increasing Caloric Contribution from Sugar-Sweetened Beverages and 100% Fruit Juices among U.S. Children and Adolescents, 1998–2004." *Pediatrics,* 2008; 121 (6):1604–1614.

60 Nestle, M. "Food Marketing and Childhood Obesity." *New England Journal of Medicine,* June 2006; 354:2527–2529.

61 Hirsch, A. R., et al. "Health Effects of Caffeine in Commercial Cola Beverages." *Alternative and Complementary Therapies,* December 2007, 298–303.

62 Fisher, J. O., et al. "Material Milk Consumption Predicts the Tradeoff Between Milk and Soft Drinks in Young Girls' Diets." *American Society for Nutritional Sciences,* 2000, 246–250.

63 He, F. J., et al. "Salt Intake Is Related to Soft Drink Consumption in Children and Adolescents." *Hypertension,* 2008; 51:629.

64 Cashdan, E. "Adaptiveness of Food Learning and Food Aversions in Children." *Anthropology of Food,* 1998; 37(4):613–632.

65 Ibid.

66 Chatoor, I. "Feeding Disorders in Infants and Toddlers: Diagnosis and Treatment." *Child & Adolescent Psychiatric Clinics of North America,* 2002; 11:163–183.

67 Chatoor, I., et al. "Failure to Thrive and Cognitive Development in Toddlers with Infantile Anorexia." *Pediatrics,* 2004; 113(5):440–447.

68 Smith, J. "Kids' Menus Are Growing Up." *Kansas City Star,* May 14, 2009. Cites report from Technomic.

69　Ibid. Cites report from NPD Group, Inc.

70　"Obesity on Kids' Menus at Top Chains." *Center for Science in the Public Interest Report,* 2008.

71　Wyatt, K. "Kids' Cooking Camps Sizzling in Popularity." Associated Press. July 11, 2008.

72　Forney, Matthew. "Scorpions for Breakfast and Snails for Dinner." *New York Times,* June 10, 2008.

73　Fisher, J. O. "Parents' Restrictive Feeding Practices are Associated with Young Girls' Negative Self-Evaluation of Eating." *American Journal of Clinical Nutrition,* 2000; 71:1054–1061.

74　Parker-Pope, T. "Six Food Mistakes Parents Make." *New York Times,* September 15, 2008.

INDEX

⌘